Early Praise for V

M000110709

"This book can help readers sort out their personal values on this intimate and inevitable subject. The first-person writing is unsparing in its argument that lack of directives, and poor ones, only lead to more confusion over the health system's rules and regulations and more suffering of patients."

— Judge, 23rd Annual Writer's Digest
Self-Published Book Awards.

"Drawing from his experiences as an emergency room physician, Dr. Kevin Haselhorst has crafted his book *Wishes to Die For* as a heartfelt and enlightened appeal that 'patients be allowed to die the way their doctors do.' His thoughtful Universal Healthcare Directive should serve as a roadmap for future discussions as we ponder how to honor our patients' dignity and divinity at the end-of-life."

— **Karen Wyatt, MD, hospice physician and author of**
What Really Matters

"In *Wishes To Die For,* Dr. Kevin Haselhorst brings his deep experience as an ER physician to the task of helping us, and those we love, die with forethought, dignity, and peacefulness."

— **Larry Dossey, MD, author of *One Mind: How Our Individual***
Mind Is Part of a Greater Consciousness and Why It Matters

"It's well worth taking this journey with the author to help us clarify our own beliefs." Excerpt from the Foreword

— **Carol Bradley Bursack, columnist and author of**
Minding Our Elders

"It's unusual to be able to tap into an emergency department physician's thinking on the topic of advance care planning. He himself seeks '"to be conscious long enough to make dying mindful, meaningful, and certain."' That's an outcome that many of us would value."

— **Deborah J. Cornwall, author of**
Things I Wished I'd Known: Cancer Caregivers Speak Out

"This book is very helpful for health care providers, patients, and families when approaching death or when people are planning for their death even when death is not imminent. The author has vast experience in this area and brings his experience, wisdom, and humor to this often-ignored task. The book was helpful to me personally and professionally and I recommend it to clients."

— **Carolyn Conger, PhD, author of *Through the Dark Forest: Transforming Your Life in the Face of Death***

"Through *Wishes To Die For*, Dr. Haselhorst poignantly demonstrates the importance of completing Healthcare Directives. Truly, end-of-life conversations begin in the heart of the person and their family prior to being addressed by a physician, hospital policy, or the government. This book shows us how to start the journey with our loved ones in the comfort of our homes."

— **Deb Lavender, Missouri State Representative**

"Brilliantly written and a book that needs to be read by many as we will all face these issues at some time. A subject that needs more attention."

— **William Tacchi, Director of Rehabilitation, Brookdale Rancho Mirage, California**

"I was afraid that your book would take me places I either did not want to be reminded of, or were just plain painful. You have been able to relieve some fear for me."

— **Charles Metz, O.D., Ph.D, Chicago, Illinois**

"Kevin's perspective helped me re-frame my views on death, as I faced my mom's passing, making the loss I was feeling less difficult to face and more meaningful to me."

— **Bren Shropshire, consultant and columnist, Healthy Solutionz, Greensboro, North Carolina**

"Since I am re-working my own living will and advance medical directives, I learned a whole lot that I didn't know, which will very much affect what I include in the new documents."

— **Paul McNeese, founder, OPA Author Services, Scottsdale, Arizona**

Wishes To Die For

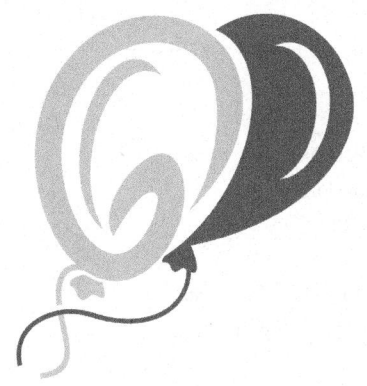

A Caregiver's Guide
to Advance Care Directives

Kevin J. Haselhorst, MD

Tranquility Publications
Scottsdale, Arizona

Best Wishes Kimberly !

Tranquility Publications
7349 N. Via Paseo Del Sur, Suite 515-257
Scottsdale, Arizona 85258
www.tranquilitypulications.com

ISBN 978-0-9915714-4-4
Cover art graciously donated by Osnat Tzadok at
www.osnatfineart.com

Cover Design Rob Wilke, Phatanium.com
Anita Jones, www.anotherjones.com
Interior Design: Michael Leclair

Publisher's Cataloging-In-Publication Data
(Prepared by The Donohue Group, Inc.)

Haselhorst, Kevin J.
   Wishes To Die For : a caregiver's guide to advance care directives /
Kevin J. Haselhorst, MD.

   pages ; cm

   Includes bibliographical references and index.
   ISBN: 978-0-9915714-4-4

   1. Advance directives (Medical care) 2. Terminal care. 3. Terminally ill--Psychology.
4. Caregivers--Psychology. I. Title.

R726.2 .H37 2016
362.17/5

**Partial proceeds support children's charities
that make heartfelt wishes come true.**

Manufactured in the United States of America

With the certainty of being right,
I dedicate this book to my parents
Martin and Mary Ann Haselhorst

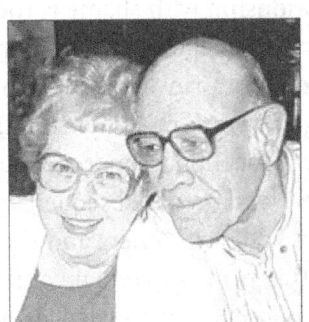

Acknowledgements

Considering the source of *Wishes To Die For*, I acknowledge the stream of consciousness that occurs while writing and seems to flow from the reservoir of messages instilled by my parents. With the parental challenge to be more Christ-like, I took to heart the dagger of their imposing words, "Shame on you." Through pointing out my flaws, Mom and Dad reflected and reiterated the inherent, undying struggle that exists between being human and indignation. Resolving interpersonal conflict can occur through contemplative writing which allows the heart and soul to speak. Reconciling personal shame leads to making peace with both parents and my own humanity in order that we all might rest in peace.

The contentious relationship with shame is rooted in childhood, reinforced by parents and can last a lifetime. Landmark Education, a personal growth and development company, provided the tools and motivation for me to shovel through layers of misunderstanding between my parents and myself. Landmark Education proposes that when the parent/child relationship is perceived as flawed, subsequent relationships tend to be doomed. True intimacy with self, others and the end of life necessitates healing and honoring this primal parental connection. Through a deep debt of gratitude to my parents, I acknowledge and apologize for faulting them as being less than perfect. Truly, they experienced and perpetuated similar deep-seated wounds that had been inflicted by their own less-than-perfect parents. Breaking my own chains of shame through forgiveness and compassion while writing *Wishes To Die For*, provided for personal growth with potential global ramifications.

From my early roots in the field of medicine as a certified nurse assistant to later becoming a senior attending physician in the Emergency Department, I have remained servant and master to many formidable nurses. As guardian angels, their eyes, ears and voices have functioned in concert to convey and raise my awareness of adding compassion to patient care. My greatest affirmation comes from peer references from nurses who stroke my ego and celebrate my aptitude. It was a nursing director who offered me my first job in an ED as an ER Tech. It was nursing staff who credentialed me at a Level I Trauma Center after moonlighting there as an Internal Medicine resident. It was charge nurses who requested I intercede on behalf of patients confronting end-of-life situations. Each of these situations culminated in my higher calling to serve patients with an appreciation of myself.

Random acts of kindness signify devoutness to the golden rule and spread a type of contagious spirituality. I catch demonstrations of this through the real lives of hospital volunteers who continually provide a safe haven for individuality through the demonstration of unconditional love. Early in my career, one of these spiritual guides sought to fill a personal and professional void in my life by suggesting a reading list that instilled awareness of the kingdom of God abiding in the heart. This key message has unlocked the heart of my humanness through Landmark Education, the heart of my spirit through the teachings of Dr. H. Brugh Joy and the heart of empowerment through the practice of yoga. These heart-centered disciplines constantly remind me to acknowledge the moment and let go.

Life is both precious and transient. In this regard, the interaction and transference that occurs in the physician/patient relationship has provided numerous life lessons throughout my career. Important answers to questions of either what or what not to do are continually related through a myriad of patients' medical complaints, treatment responses and invaluable feedback. Patients epitomize the notion that certain situations are insufferable when illness becomes tenuous, leading to uncertainty regarding the entire healthcare system. Through the art of listening—intently while appreciating that there is always another side to the story—my practice of medicine has shifted from caring for *patients* to understanding *people.*

For alchemy to occur while mixing the pseudoscience of spirituality with the science of medicine, the magic wand of an editor necessarily adds distinction, clarity and consecration to the written word. It also helps if the editor has a master's degree in counseling, skills at life coaching and is a lifelong friend. That labor of love as gifted by my devoted editor—Steven Nissenbaum—has been the saving grace of *Wishes To Die For* from its conception, throughout its gestation and now birthing process. Notably and nobly assisting in the editing process were Laura Markowitz, Ethel Burstein, Judy Pyanowski, Dennis Rose, Gary Behrman, Steven Dina, Barbara Carson and Glenn Swain. Each of them challenged me to redefine my intention and refine my message while acknowledging my passion.

Positioned behind the personal computer screen of this manuscript was the high-tech genius Rob Wilke. He was ready, willing and able to make my words and ideas pop professionally, visually and ethereally. If this book was another version of the film *Toy Story*, then I would play the role of Woody and Rob would be Buzz Lightyear. Together, we support imagination that leads to empowerment, complete with a rocket booster to infinity and beyond. The icing on the cake occurred when Rob instinctively found the *Tree of Life* by acclaimed artist, Osnat Tzadok. Osnat generously offered her brilliant masterpiece to grace the cover of *Wishes To Die For* and showcase its message.

While I can never truly know the extraordinary gift that people represent in my life, I am overwhelmed by how they show up during times of need. One of those times was while writing this book. From random passengers next to me on airplanes to people seated next to me at work or at dinner, their positive energy has infused this endeavor. When beginning to write, an elderly patient frustrated by the "system" managed to find redeeming value in our conversation. After being discharged from the ED—and with the use of a cane—she made a valiant effort to return to ensure that I was aware that she knew I was extraordinary. The universe constantly teaches that support for one another is a natural and astounding phenomenon. I acknowledge and celebrate this universal support in the creation of *Wishes To Die For*.

TABLE OF WISHES

FOREWORD... xi

INTRODUCTION xiii

I: APPEAL FOR ADVANCE CARE DIRECTIVES
WISH 1: Self-Determination 2
WISH 2: Self-Respect.. 9
WISH 3: Self-Prescribed Dignity....................................... 16
WISH 4: Self-Awareness.. 22
WISH 5: Self-Restraint Regarding Healthcare 30
WISH 6: Self-Deference to the Heart-Center 36

II. COMMENCEMENT OF ADVANCED CARE DIRECTIVES
WISH 7: Pre-Counsel and Guidance................................ 43
WISH 8: Pre-End-of-Life Plan 50
WISH 9: Pre-Wish for Peace 56
WISH 10: Pre-Stamp Three Coins in the Fountain 63
WISH 11: Pre-Ordain Healthcare Proxy............................ 66
WISH 12: Pre-Meditate Critical Thinking.......................... 71

III. PREAMBLE TO ADVANCE CARE DIRECTIVES
WISH 13: Co-Mingle Denial with Consideration............. 86
WISH 14: Co-Establish Consternation with Constitution........... 91
WISH 15: Co-Ordinate Flexibility with Rigor Mortis..................... 94
WISH 16: Co-Opt Close-Mindedness with Listening 100
WISH 17: Co-Habitat Challenges with Centeredness................. 104
WISH 18: Co-Conspire Empathy, Euthanasia
            and Exceptionalism 107

WISH 19: Co-Elaborate Chosen over Conquered........................ 116
WISH 20: Co- Join End-Stage with Predetermination............... 122

IV. ENACTMENT OF ADVANCE CARE DIRECTIVES

WISH 21: Pro-Life Disposition... 130
WISH 22: Pro-Life Survival of the Fittest................................ 137
WISH 23: Pro-Life Anger Management 142
WISH 24: Pro-Choice Evolution... 145
WISH 25: Pro-Choice Survival Rule of Threes......................... 147
WISH 26: Pro-Choice in the Context of Hope 152
WISH 27: Pro-End-of-Life Revelation 159
WISH 28: Pro-End-of-Life Survival Instinct Unplugged 164
WISH 29: Pro-End-of-Life Resolution 168

V. DELIVERANCE THROUGH ADVANCE CARE DIRECTIVES

WISH 30: Neo-Life upon Crossing the Finish Line..................... 176
WISH 31: Neo-Logic for Integrating Good and Evil 181
WISH 32: Neo-Realization of Death as a Blessing..................... 185
WISH 33: Neo-Concept of Omega Care................................. 190
WISH 34: Neo-Alignment of Directives with Desires................. 195
WISH 35: Neo-Conservative Non-verbal Compassion 199
WISH 36: Neo-Horizon of a Promised Land............................ 207
WISH 37: Neo-Nuance of Self-Validation............................... 211
WISH 38: Neo-Insurgence of Resurrection 213

APPENDIXES

I: Note to Mom 223
II: Note to Dad.. 225
III: Will to Die... 227
IV: Universal Healthcare Directive 229

ABOUT THE AUTHOR 231

KEYNOTE SPEAKER 232

Foreword

"Code Blue!" A voice cries out in the Emergency Department. "Is there a doctor who can 'tube' a patient in Cardiac Cath Lab?"

With these first lines of *Wishes To Die For: A Caregiver's Guide to Advance Care Directives*, Dr. Kevin J. Haselhorst prepares readers for a journey that will help them clarify their personal views about what constitutes life.

What decisions do you want made for you as you approach your final days, hours or minutes, or even earlier if an incapacitating event alters your ability to make your own medical decisions even temporarily? Does your spouse know what you'd want? Do your other family members? If you have not made your wishes clear, in written form, often what the medical team may be required to do could conflict with what you or your family wants done or not done. Why? Because without written guidance, once you or your loved one are in the care of medical personnel their medical oath and directive will prevail.

Dr. Haselhorst knows about this subject from the perspective of a compassionate physician. In *"Wishes"* he describes his own internal battle to balance his training as a doctor who "'cures at all costs'" with his patients' desires. Through his book, Haselhorst encourages us, as potential patients, to examine our right to decide how, and under what circumstances, we will be allowed to die a natural death.

Haselhorst builds a solid case that a document expressing our end-of-life desires should be fluid, changing with our age, our health and our own fluctuating point of view. The treatment that we would choose when we are 35 years old may be vastly different from the treatment we'd choose at age 80.

He writes, "I cannot remember the last time that I wished for a feeding tube, dialysis or ventilator." Haselhorst is not denigrating life-saving treatments. He is simply stressing that we must continually update our health directive so that it reflects our current wishes.

Haselhorst challenges us to examine what we would want as our lives evolve. Treatments that increase our chances for survival may be a correct choice under some circumstances. But there often comes a time in our lives where less medical intervention is in our best interest. Unless our current wishes are made known to our health providers and family, we may not be able to choose the manner in which our life comes to a close.

While reading the book I underlined, highlighted, and placed colored tabs on pages so that I could remember the most vital information and pass it along. Before long, I realized Haselhorst's words must be read in the context of the book in order to reveal their full meaning.

Haselhorst believes strongly that people have a right to change their minds about end-of-life care right up to their last breath. To address this belief, he has designed a wristband similar to the ubiquitous Livestrong Foundation wristband. Haselhorst's wrist band is bright yellow and embossed with the words "Alpha Care" on one side meaning that the patient wishes doctors to keep trying all possible treatments to keep him or her alive. The reverse side is a subdued blue and embossed with the words "'Omega Care'" indicating the patient's wish to be allowed a natural death. With a twist of the wrist band a patient can communicate his or her current feelings on whether or not to use life extending treatments.

Haselhorst sums up his message with the words, "Dying with dignity is only realized through the empowerment attained from engagement of the patient."

This thought-provoking book offers you a method of engagement and a map to that empowerment. I strongly recommend that you take this opportunity to learn more about exerting as much control as possible over your own final experience.

By Carol Bradley Bursack,
columnist and author of *Minding Our Elders*

Introduction

Doctors don't die the way their patients do. Most doctors lead full lives, retire and vow to never again step foot in a hospital. Many elderly patients frequent Emergency Departments and are subsequently admitted to hospitals and extended-care institutions. While practicing emergency medicine, I help facilitate end-of-life choices that seem to disrespect the prevailing wish to die at home. Patients have an opportunity to express their end-of-life wishes through Advance Care Directives. However, these documents frequently and heedlessly result in life-saving treatment that bombards their lives with additional suffering.

Caregivers rarely consider the consequences of their choices regarding their loved ones' end-of-life care. *Wishes To Die For* provides a type of internal emotional support system for caregivers who struggle with the moral dilemma posed by Confucius: "Don't do unto others what you don't want others to do to you." Introspection and forethought comprise *A Caregiver's Guide to Advance Care Directives*. The intention to *pull the plug* on myself personally necessitates good conscience overriding best practice in medicine. By demonstrating a strategy to preempt standard critical care with heartfelt critical thinking, I give those dying and caregivers permission to experience the end of life as a blessing rather than an emergency.

Wishes To Die For attempts to balance the hopes and dreams of staying alive with the practical and spiritual certainty essential for advance care planning. As the book cover suggests, this is an impressionistic work. Impressionism captures stories amid activities of daily life with unusual angles of light, portraying the here and now that fleets with time. My practice of medicine involves gathering information and making notes for future reference. This diary of sorts assimilates these scribbled messages and hewed pieces into a mosaic of a tree. Each branch is a tributary and expression of a wish that sprouts individual leaves. In conjunction with each branch is an invisible root of self-preservation that requires excavation and examination.

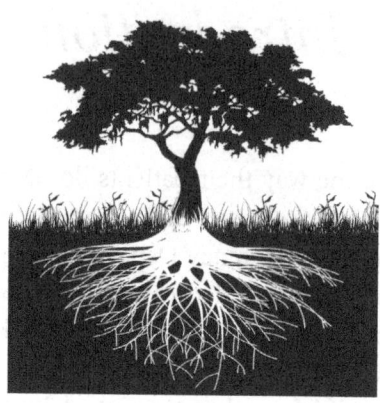

Trees eventually die, but they provide vivid examples of life cycles and adaptation. Through their xylem and phloem, trees repeatedly take from the earth and give back to the universe unconsciously and unconditionally. Trees sway in splendor, cast shadows and remain indifferent to their own purpose and existence. Nonetheless, they drop leaves like hints, providing awareness that living entities can coexist admirably amid the forces of nature through both fortitude and receptivity to the changing seasons. Nature never calls us to endure situations that are not humanly possible in attempts to live forever. Human nature concedes having to confront and mourn the loss of a tree—people we love dying and ourselves dying.

Reconciling human nature with Mother Nature remains conflicted. What we wish for and what mothers generally sanction is dependent on them being deliberate, selective and heart-warming. Similar to soul food, Mom's stew warms the cockles of my heart. Mom knows that a multitude of ingredients taste good, but not when they are haphazardly lumped together. In the same say, the stew served at the end of life is potentially measured and concocted through Advance Care Directives. *Wishes To Die For* offers the fixings but is not an actual formula. It provides personalized spiritual rudiments for individuals to accept or reject as provisions, to facilitate discussions and to create possible documentations for end-of-life care.

Most people become conscious of dying when emotions are heightened by a visit to the Emergency Department, especially when registration clerks inquire about having Advance Care Directives. Thoughts of dying lead to introspection; wishes emerge from introspection. A subconscious, heart-centered awareness is the source that allows us to be connected spiritually, emotionally and universally. Spirituality naturally guides life's path and serves as a refuge from suffering often triggered by emotions. *Wishes To Die For* offers a mixed bag of thought-provoking emotions from which final wishes might be selected—those determined to be paramount to an individual and rising to that individual's convictions. Channeling these emotions becomes the spiritual foundation that is both necessary and lacking from current Advance Care Directives.

Many incidents that amount to atrocities at life's end and very few of these crimes against humanity are openly and willingly discussed. While people prefer speaking about subjects they are passionate about, typically, this does not include their personal passion and death. The message of this book is a memo regarding wishes to live by. Its impetus will hopefully create a paradigm shift in this area of life: Never put off until tomorrow what you can do today. Live today as you wish to be remembered, remaining relevant in life and not left to die unconsciously. Consciously accepting what life has to offer in the moment and then releasing it as time passes supports the fundamental inclusion and connection to the circle of life.

Having put forth my wishes, I realize they are not unlike most people's. This awareness might offer a compromise in physician/patient relationship, paying homage to the golden rule while declaring a truce to crusades often waged at the end of life. Patients might actually be allowed to die the way their doctors do, physicians could more readily treat patients the way they would wish to be treated. Loving one another over expecting more from loved ones seems reasonable and rational in regard to the end of life. Changing the paradigm of dying with dignity from being an isolated journey to becoming more of a collective enterprise will require a heartfelt appreciation of universal truths and wishes.

This book positions me as narrator and spokesman for end-of-life conversations through the guideline of a Universal Healthcare Directive (Appendix IV). This futurist concept is not an actual document, but a spiritual framework from which to make medical decisions. Dignity is not a medical word, yet there are attempts to squeeze its round peg into the square hole of a hospital room. We need to think outside of this box and away from the fear that overshadows death and dying. Wishes can seize a person's values from the grips of fear while using them to proclaim a significant cause from which to die. Today, most people will die in fear. *Wishes To Die For* encourages people to prioritize their lives, making the end of life conscious, manageable and heart-centered.

PART I

...

Appeal For
Advance Care Directives

WISH 1:

Self-Determination

"**C**ODE BLUE!" A voice cries out in the Emergency Department. "Is there a doctor who can 'tube' a patient in the Cardiac Cath Lab?"

On your mark . . . get set . . . go! In the blink of an eye I immediately clear my to-do list and dart down the hospital corridors to the CC Lab like a well-trained athlete. Swiping my name tag at door sensors along the way, I am struck that being an emergency medicine physician provides me immediate, unparalleled access to the inner recesses of others' lives. They trust me with their lives and the challenges that surround the end of life. Jumping these hurdles requires self-determination in figuring out what is going on with, around and inside patients.

In life-threatening emergencies, there is rarely time to stop and question patients: "What would you like us to do?" "Did you plan for this moment?" or "Let's sit down and weigh in on all your hopes and dreams,"—so their every wish is understood, respected and carried out. The truth is, those questions need to be asked earlier—much earlier—when people are in the prime of life and not gasping for breath. But few patients consciously prepare themselves for dying.

EM physicians attend to people near death while on guard, internally, often sharing the same helplessness and confusion they face regarding life-and-death issues. How would I feel if my life hung in the balance? What would I want done in these situations? Emergency Medicine physicians learn from the first day of training to always expect the unexpected. These years of trial by fire in managing life-threatening situations teach valuable lessons that provide both insight and perspective.

I enter the vented surgical suite and greet "the Colonel." He is struggling to breathe, his Chronic Obstructive Pulmonary Disease (COPD) flaring in conjunction with an evolving heart attack. He is expected to lie flat, but this is a real struggle as he has lost a lung to cancer. Cardiac catheterization involves threading a catheter from the groin to the blocked heart artery with the intention of opening the vessel and restoring blood flow to the heart muscle. The Colonel is exhausted, but he does not wish to be placed on a ventilator. He knows once he is on "that machine," it will keep him alive indefinitely and limit his ability to maintain any sense of control. The Colonel has reached a breaking point. He is ready to call it quits.

The cardiac team is in place and ready to proceed with the procedure. Delays risk damage to the Colonel's heart. There had already been a critical delay in diagnosing his evolving heart attack, as he did not complain of any chest pain and his EKG was overlooked. Nevertheless, his blood work indicated a heart attack. Here, at our certified Chest Pain Center, there is a 90-minute window after patients arrive to open the blocked vessels that cause heart attacks. The clock is ticking.

Literally, the Colonel is drowning from lack of oxygen. He knows his time is limited. When I reach the Colonel, he is on the cellphone to his wife in California—"I don't want any more of this bullshit. I want them to leave me alone."

Under the Patient's Bill of Rights, a patient has the right you have the right to know their treatment options and take part in decisions involving their care. Patients have the right to ask about the pros and cons of any treatment. One option is no treatment at all. However, these rights are set aside when patients are incompetent or in an emergency situations. In emergencies, physicians act in the best interest of the patient with best standard practice.

In the control room off the surgical suite, the on-call cardiologist is focused on the medical crisis, not the patient. That's logical. Her duty is to respond to the emergency, not to determine the competency of the patient. That is my job. The Colonel may have been flustered initially, but he seems to be making sense now. What began as a little stick to his groin—now involves inserting a PVC pipe through his vocal cords and placing him on life support. He appears to be aware of the consequences of not having the cardiac catheterization and says he is ready to die.

I realize I am no longer being called to intubate this patient, but rather, to negotiate a settlement between treating the patient and honoring his self-determination. His wishes loud and clear, but is he competent? Should we respect them? Am I a witness to a potential lawsuit or perhaps a party in a malpractice case? The proverbial hot potato is tossed in my lap.

My decision-making has been impacted by the thorough training previously undergone by all physicians. There is an algorithm for every procedure taught in medical school. But there are no algorithms to shock the physician's heart and convert it from the fast-paced demands of saving lives to the aberrant rhythms that allow for death.

Each heart has an inherent pacemaker that is apt to go awry with time, insult or injury. Technology can rewire the heart with a pacemaker embedded under the skin or pacer pads on top of the chest, stimulating heartbeats. Periodically, the pacemaker is "interrogated" to assess how well it is functioning. As external pacemakers, doctors monitor and intervene when hearts race, miss beats or go extended periods without beating. Absent of any protocols for knowing when it may be time to cease treatment, doctors rarely withhold those interventions necessary for life. They are reluctant to allow the inherent pacemaker of the heart to determine when it should stop beating.

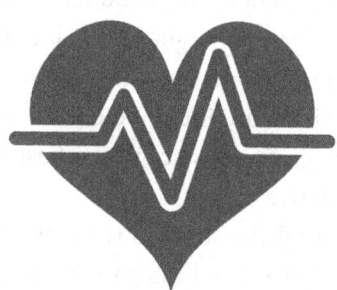

The cardiologist is quick to step aside; I remain ringside. The Colonel is pursed-lip breathing as if attempting to blow out candles on his birthday cake. Fueled by his resolve, his lungs expand like bellows flaming a fire. Standing back from this ceremonial rite of passage, I realize that people have to blow out their own candles for their wish to come true.

I am handed the cellphone by the Colonel and confirm that his wife supports his wishes. In relief and celebration, I place a reassuring hand on the Colonel's shoulder and call out, "Nurse, get this man a double shot of Ativan." Subtle whoops and cheers permeate the room as if I had just bought a round of Ativan shots for everyone. My hand resting on his shoulder offers a pat on the back for a job well done.

Out of the depths of his misery, the Colonel's self-preservation was aligned with self-determination—maintaining control over his destiny rather than holding onto his life. I admired his tenacity. In addition, he was blessed to have a wife supportive of his intention and a doctor willing to listen. With his suffering eased and awareness of this man's dignity shining forth, it seemed another voice was crying from above: *Let my people go, so they may serve Me* (Exodus 9:1).

As a physician, I am obliged to pursue measures that preserve life. The Patient Self-Determination Act of 1990 provides the right for healthcare decisions to be personal and protected. Patients can accept or refuse treatment and document their wishes in Advance Care Directives. It allows for patients to sign-out against medical advice as long as they are competent. Self-determination reassures patients, but is by no means a safeguard against obligations to save a life. When self-determination appears destructive to the person, the Good Samaritan law rescinds all rights.

A much younger Native American man, Daniel—presumably had the same self-determination as the Colonel—but arrived in the ED unresponsive. He was an alcoholic with liver disease. However, this time he was not in a stupor from too much alcohol, but from a high ammonia level in his system, lulling his brain to sleep. When the liver is diseased, it fails to break down ammonia. His kidneys were also failing, so a liver transplant would not be considered. I was certain Daniel would die of liver disease, but I was uncertain as to whether he was ready and determined to die at this moment.

Daniel's sister was at his bedside and obviously preferred I do everything to keep him alive. The usual treatment would be to admit him to the hospital, administer some Lactulose to bind the ammonia, remove it from his system and raise his awareness of dying. The prospects seemed self-defeating rather than self-determined. Obviously, Daniel did not arrive in the ED of his own volition. His sister finally managed to gain control over his life. I felt compelled to take Daniel's side in this presumed sibling squabble, not allowing his sister to have full reign over Daniel's self-determination.

What would Daniel do? In a roundabout way I began to question his sister. Did Daniel ever try to stop drinking? Was he aware of the consequences of his drinking? She replied that he never intended to stop drinking. He had buried several cousins and a brother who were alcoholics; he knew where he was headed.

I ascribe to the belief that actions speak louder than words. Since Daniel could not speak, it was not a stretch to think he preferred to be at home drinking rather than having a hose shoved up his nose to administer Lactulose. The Lactulose would lower his ammonia level, but the miserable side effect is ongoing diarrhea. Daniel was peacefully sleeping at the moment.

In the wake of having to re-intubate a similar patient with end-stage liver disease being treated in the Intensive Care Unit, I could see where Daniel was headed. This patient had varicose veins in his esophagus that were bleeding profusely. His clotting factors that are normally produced by the liver were missing in action. As quickly as blood and clotting factors were being infused, this patient was disgustingly spewing blood from both ends. Nevertheless, his wife was determined to have us save his life.

In advocating for Daniel's self-determination, I risked my professional obligation and went out on a limb with his sister to discuss options. The more I brought Daniel's behavior into the conversation, the more she agreed that he would not wish any medical intervention I had to offer. Rather than pursuing unnecessary treatment in the hospital, I asked her to consider a hospice consult and simply allow him to remain comfortable. However, the hospice nurse was skeptical of accepting Daniel without my first treating him "appropriately." I was certain I was respecting his wishes and right to an unspoken self-determination.

The relationship between self-determination and a physician's duty presented itself when a recent widow, Esther, was brought into the Emergency Department with a head gash. Three days after her husband's death, grieving, weak and dizzy from not eating, she fell and hit her head on the bathroom sink. Her stepdaughter heard the thump and went to assist her. When she saw blood, she drove her in to the emergency department.

This sweet woman made a gash in my psyche about how I treat people. I struggled between treating her as a grieving person and my obligation to care for her as a patient. She inspired me to pause in my duty, center in our conversation and shift my awareness. The pause was easy. While simultaneously rubbing her head to both cleanse the wound and calm her mind, I stapled her anesthetized wound while dwelling on her evaluation. Should I run her through various tests that most elderly patients have ordered following a syncopal episode and head injury? This could include CT scan of the brain, blood work and an EKG in consideration of other reasons for her fall. Maybe I would allow self-determination to address what was most important to her regarding her care.

In the desolate moment her mind was focused on the question: "How is someone supposed to grieve?" I suggested that perhaps some of her grief had to be released for her to resume eating. I also shared my own recipe for containing grief after realizing the benefits from participating in restorative yoga classes; ideally, it restores what may be lost. The practice of yoga unites students with the divine; it connects us to our own divine nature and perhaps the beloved within in this sacred space. Restorative yoga potentially nurtures emptiness by replenishing the person's spirit and energy.

With this refreshing outlook, her facial expression visibly shifted. The idea of using grief to restore, refuel and nurture herself seemed more palatable than allowing grief to let her body become its punching bag. She gladly took to heart the "Popsicle" I offered. With her stepdaughter's blessing, we averted any further evaluation. I mentioned I was becoming more aware of dignity being stripped from people while they are treated as patients.

On second thought, I phoned her the next day and was surprised to hear her answer the phone in a youthful tone. I expressed possibly being remiss in not giving her the complete ED work-up. Would she like to return and have further testing done? She assured me she had eaten that day and was feeling significantly better, though she felt somewhat humiliated. She had told no one about her ED visit and remembered my conversation regarding the indignation that sometimes surrounds patients in dire straits. In retrospect, she could not help but wonder what it must have been like for her husband to have endured his years of suffering and hospitalizations. If she had a role in it, we mutually agreed in there being little merit in persecuting those who suffer.

What the Colonel, Daniel and Esther each want is self-determination. The Colonel's was explicit, Daniel's was implied and Esther's was shared decision-making. In essence, self-determination means this is your life to do with as you wish. My role in self-determination is not to assume responsibility for patients' decisions, but rather to help facilitate the process. Many patients present with a medical complaint and an ulterior motive. My professional determination seeks to arrive at a diagnosis and discern their ulterior motives. Ulterior motives are people's wishes.

From the medicolegal perspective, it is always safer to keep patients alive. Although people have the right to die, the problem with self-determination is the perception that people in their right minds rarely choose to die. Any wish to die needs to be well-thought-out and expressed through a pre-determined Advance Care Directives. Sadly, many Advance Care Directives seem to circumvent the prospect of dying and what it means to be treated humanely with dignity. When self-determination exists in wishes to avert death, how does anyone hope to retain self-respect during the process of dying?

WISH 2:

Self-Respect

The purpose of end-of-life conversations is to encourage awareness and respect for the process of dying. Awareness, reconciliation and acceptance of any apparent medical condition are how we discover our resilience, resolve and self-respect. There is a time to live and a time to die. Might a wish to die actually include self-respect as a guide and goal for the journey? As we embark upon life and proceed "over the hill," it is natural to look ahead and be curious about what awaits.

In the past, dying was considered a natural part of life. It would come to everyone sooner or later; the key was meeting it with acceptance or denial. When did dying become so stressful? While there is a time to live and a time to die, little consideration is paid to how and when to die. Many people want to live forever, having a childish superstition about death and dying: If I do not think about it, it will not happen.

Stress naturally escalates in this never-ending quest to survive. I observe many patients experiencing death as a catastrophic emergency. Yet by definition, an emergency is something unexpected; death is expected. With preparation and planning, dying is anticipated and addressed. A clear plan brings certainty to crisis: here is the anticipated event, and here is the plan that is put in place to address it. Imagine your response if someone collapsed on the street in front of you. The average person with CPR training knows to call 911 and begin compressions. They are called to action as part of their training. An untrained person does not have a plan, so they hesitate, panic or do nothing.

The purpose of Advance Care Directives is to have a plan in place so others may respect your wishes. Doctors and nurses encourage people to complete or at least think about Advance Care Directives, but few patients, caregivers and relatives take time to truly consider what is respectful for the dying. People tend to believe death will not happen any time soon. However, self-respect that emerges out of respect for the nature of death inherent to humanity requires more attention than wishful thinking.

As an EM physician, I am torn between comforting dying patients and providing them with options to live longer. Astounding advancements in technology and medical science ensure patients can be kept alive indefinitely. As recently as 20 years ago a doctor might turn to the family and proclaim, "We've done all we can; it's time to say good-bye." The patient could then breathe a sigh of relief and let go.

Now families look at their loved one, who is hooked up to multiple devices that breathe for them, administer medication and provide nutrition. They are not sure what to do. Is death imminent? Is this what he wanted? And sadly, in our increasingly litigious society, am I incurring possible legal action by not providing more extreme care before patients are allowed to die.

We are strongly encouraged to reject the inevitability of death. "Not now!" we protest. In the famous last words of Queen Victoria, "There are several things I want to arrange." Like a personal journal, *Wishes To Die For* presents an opportunity to reflect upon heartfelt wishes in order to purposefully arrange affairs. Wishes proclaim our heart's desires and self-examination of them garners self-respect. When our desires are written down in a well-organized plan, it is essentially becomes the same exercise that involves connecting the dots with the realization of a clear, self-serving image of a directive.

The first barrier is accepting death as inevitable. But there are other factors. When illness, injury and aging bring us closer to death, self-respect often breaks down. Peace of mind quickly plummets, creating shame. I often see this response in stroke patients who suddenly become stripped of their functionality, independence and self-respect. The best remedy for shame is dignity. Accordingly, every life has value; every person deserves respect. Ideally, each one of us has the ability to master self-respect throughout life, particularly while dying. Too often, when people declare, "I'm ready to die," their statement is dismissed as preposterous. They cannot mean it; they are unstable or just plain crazy. What self-respecting person chooses to die, creating a quagmire?

Dying is a barren experience. Therefore, it is incumbent on us to shield ourselves with self-affirming virtues and defenses that raise our self-esteem. Only when our intentions and actions have been validated by our heart and soul, can we hope to stand strong amid adversity. Every wish becomes another building block to our fortress of self-respect amid the forces that shame us while dying. Naturally, we must confront our fearful inner child who instinctively rejects darkness and the unknown. Our adult self recognizes the need to find out what lies ahead and make informed decisions for our own protection.

Dying brings disorder into lives; it strikes at the heart of all our fears. We are apt to make choices in the moment that would normally never make sense to us at other times. Being emotional is understandable, yet self-respect for ourselves insists we maintain control. Self-respect mirrors self-control.

Nevertheless, people do panic. Physicians bent on prolonging life implement procedures with the assumption that the patient does not wish to die. The fanfare we confront at the end of life surges like a stadium filled with Brits bellowing out "God save the Queen!" Typically, our petition insists everyone deserves a stay of execution. We all deserve to be blessed and granted longevity; let the physician be aggressive. For those at center-stage, there is little choice in this subjugation. Dying potentially becomes abusive when patients feel compelled to oblige the duties of others. The truth is that dying needs to be about respecting the wishes of those who are on the journey, not in attempting to please everyone else.

I participate in the dying process in one of several roles: advocate, persecutor or savior, depending on perspective. When the Colonel was dying, I assessed the situation, judged him competent and advocated for his wishes. In a different situation with a healthier patient, I might determine that the patient's wishes either do not respect life or the reality of the situation. Then I may become the persecutor masked as the Good Samaritan. Sometimes I am lucky and God intervenes in saving a life, with me receiving the credit.

I view my medical career as a ministry in cultivating and making a difference in people's lives while restoring self-respect. With each intervention I question whether I am respecting or diminishing my patient's capacity. In prolonging someone's life, might I be perpetuating suffering? Does a particular treatment help or hinder patients in coming to terms with their spiritual and/or physical natures? Confusion and indecision cloud judgment in the face of death. Interestingly enough, studies have shown that most of what was previously outlined in Advanced Cardiac Life Support is actually detrimental to patients. ACLS has been whittled down extensively. Might we apply the same methodology to Advance Care Directives?

When time is muscle in the heat of the moment, what often seems rote to physicians is to strong-arm patients into falling in line or risk death. Typically, patients give informed consent in the presence of the veiled threat, "Do or die." Opting to go against medical advice can also carry implied consequences such as, "If you don't do this, you may die and go to hell." Taking undue risks with our lives can threaten our salvation. "Damned if you do and dammed if you don't" is often the dilemma many patients confront both during and particularly at the end of life. During a medical crisis, there may be little time or consideration that affords self-respect.

While gasping for breath, a 99-year-old man with worsening congestive heart failure was unable to answer any questions. His wife was upfront about not placing him on a ventilator; he would have allowed for anything to help him breathe. The patient was immediately given medication to lower his blood pressure and a diuretic to help the kidneys release fluid, along with continuous oxygen and mild sedation. He soon fell into what appeared to be a peaceful slumber; at times, he stopped breathing.

When I checked on him again, both the nurse and his wife were taking turns yelling at him to, "Breathe, breathe, breathe!" It is not unusual for a nurse to encourage a patient to breathe while waking from sedation, yet this situation was deeply disturbing. Was this patient allowed to determine his last breath or was the decision dependent upon another person's command? Feeling much angst I blurted out, "I don't think we are supposed to be yelling at him." This yelling became a wake-up call and I found my internal voice yelling back, "What the hell are we doing?" I no longer cared to associate with the type of medical practice that lacks reverence for the time to die.

After this situation I considered completing a fellowship in Palliative Medicine or perhaps working with hospice patients. However, I soon realized treating people with reverence is not dependent on any medical specialty that I might practice. Any self-respecting physician would offer self-respect for all patients.

My internal yelling soon diminished into mutterings about wrongdoings at the end of life. There was much more to this conversation that I did not recognize and people were not discussing. While adoring staff frequently say, "You're pretty good with these conversations," I mostly feel inadequate. As a physician who is called on to save lives, how might I encourage people to have wishes to die for in anticipation of their own day of reckoning?

The recent uproar about assembling "death panels" generated much blasphemy: How dare people talk to someone about dying? I was ecstatic that we would finally begin to talk about dying sooner than in the chaos of the Emergency Department. Unfortunately, the conversation quickly deteriorated into cost-saving measures rather than a dignity-sparing rationale. Some dimwitted people thwarted the conversation, believing death panels devalue people.

It's easy to become distracted by special interest groups; however, my personal interest was to spearhead and cultivate a personalized death panel conversation. What would it be like to defend my life in front of this panel? Wait, I would also be the person conducting the panel. Decidedly, I would have to grapple with both sides of the discussion, but what resources would guide the discussion? Patients would expect me to be the expert, but there are no medical textbooks on how to die respectfully.

Prior to beginning any type of outreach program or discussion on these issues, assessment of what is going on inside individuals and within the healthcare system needs to be earnestly weighed before any words of wisdom emerge. The immediate call to save a life inherently implies that death is wrong. Death will rarely be viewed as acceptable until death is considered a natural process and respectable option; something we can live with and take to our graves. This perspective involves rewiring our conscience with more respect given to the process of dying. While the outreach of palliative medicine is to provide self-respect for patients, I perceive the foundation for dignity beginning in preventive medicine.

It became clear that I needed to write a book as a basis for discerning potential wishes that provided insights and agendas for death panel discussions. My goal was to break down what is specifically frightening to people about death, debunk the widespread belief that death equates with failure and to shirk the duty of defying death at all cost. From my experience, problems are never solved when issues are buried amidst defense mechanisms. I wanted to move my discussion beyond the stages Elisabeth Kübler-Ross outlines in her work, *On Death and Dying.*[1]

As end-of-life wishes are often buried underneath desires to be free of pain and illness, I view wishes as being the root to spawn self-respect. In general, current literature on death and dignity, along with advance care planning, state a similar message: Know your wishe—declare them —document them. It all seems so personal and auspicious. Could I really know what I wish for while dying? Can I really create a document that enlists self-respect? The dignity I was reaching for was actually a higher realization of self.

Rev. Dr. Michele Medrano, a Religious Science minister, spoke to my objective and assignment. She remarked that her courage to stand before the congregation and preach her message reflected her willingness to go first. In the spotlight, she appreciated her higher realization of self. Extrapolating her words as the message I needed to hear, I concluded that my higher realization of self occurred while writing. In composing *Wishes To Die For*, I realized the courage necessary to going first along with being able to practice what I preach.

When I began writing, I was often questioned about my reference material. Any competent writer and doctor compiles research from published data. I sheepishly replied I was writing the book from an inside reference and life experience. Having the perspective of the dying person as *wounded child*, I appreciated the archetype of my own *wounded child* yearning for self-respect. I realized this child experiences oppression and shame on a deeper level, similar to when people are dying. This child's feelings became the basis of my writing and thread for connecting words with understanding, applying empathy to end-of life conversations.

I examined my *inner child's* personal wounds when I volunteered to be a Phoenix Valley Big Brother. Poignantly, my Little Brother testified, "Since I met you, I no longer cry at night." Years later, he wrote a winning essay titled, "Why my Big Brother is Best," a heartfelt endorsement of my metamorphosis from *wounded child* to *wound healer.*

Why I am one of the few authors to write a book on dying with self-respect stems from a child certifying his "big brother is best" and from my belief that the best is yet to come from inside. With personal reflection, a spiritual connection and some skill at writing, self-respect is what presented the opportunity to set an example of bringing self-fulfilling wishes to my Advance Care Directive.

While self-respect increases with integrity to an intention, dignity promotes the need to take action. When expectations become overwhelming there is a tendency to become distracted by rationalizations or by making excuses for misgivings, mishaps, missteps and missed opportunities; thus, missing the mark of dignity. When all of life is said and done, medicated and treated, what would we give for the opportunity to have a crystal ball to predict the future? *Wishes To Die For* provides the opportunity to dust off the proverbial crystal ball and gaze into the future with additional clarity before life-threatening situations blur the image of dignity.

WISH 3:

Self-Prescribed Dignity

Dignity is telltale of a life lived well. Even as I aspire to live with dignity, will someone tell me when I attain dignity or will I need to tell myself?

Few people nowadays reflect on what it means to die with dignity. Abhorrently, "death with dignity" has exclusively come to mean physician-assisted suicide. Dying with dignity actually envisions the brilliance of a person heading into the light. By fearing the presumed darkness of the afterlife, most people rely on procrastination, wishful thinking and blind chance. Failing to plan ahead leads to faltering while dying—losing all self-respect.

Dying with self-respect dignifies the process. Friends and relatives often comfort themselves by repeating the phrase, "He died with dignity," as if that makes everything OK. Yes, dying with dignity would preferably be a given, but what does this mean?

The reality is that during any shift in the Emergency Department, I observe patients on the brink of death rolled into the ED without a stitch of clothing. Patients at the end of their ropes are tied down with tubes and lines invading every part of their bodies as they lie injured, wounded beyond recognition, wondering what became of their lives. Are they being treated with respect and consideration? Are their wishes being carried out in this moment of crisis? I see patients struggling to hang on regardless of the cost; steadfast in their desire not to let go, accompanied by tearful relatives' appeals and prayers to raise Lazarus from the dead.

In anticipation of death, dignity might give rise to a common-sense approach that insists nothing be done other than providing comfort for the patient. My heart aches for the countless end-stage cancer patients and cardiac-crippled patients rushed through the ED entrance with one rescuer pushing oxygen through a bag, another doing chest compressions and someone else recording the patient's plight. Paramedics voice, "Sorry Doc. This wasn't supposed to happen."

Like love and gratitude, dignity is a deep-seated emotion that exists as a noun but acts like a verb. Articulating what dignity means when words provide an inadequate definition presents a dilemma. Consequently, dignity becomes lost in conversations that are nebulous and difficult to discuss. The mindset of dignity dares me to proceed forward, while the fear of death holds me back.

Each of us has one shot at this life and wants to get it right. We seek affirmation from others that we are doing the right thing, hoping to receive accolades for a life lived well. We sign-in and register at the entrance of the Emergency Department hoping to live right and be treated by the doctor who will get it right. When it comes to life and death, it is better to be safe than sorry. "Right" sides with life and "sorry" sides with death. There is no dignity in not doing things right. Therefore, I have come to define dignity as "the certainty of being right."

Combining the certainty of death with *the certainty of being right* strengthens feeling "right" when it is time to die. In effect, bringing dignity back into the conversation may mean that I am not resuscitated when it is my time to die. That unique, timely combination of certainty and courage supports dignity. Instead of giving in to blind panic, emotions can center on conviction and resolution.

Dignity and feeling right is on the line at each juncture of doing the right thing. When the certainty of being right is dependent upon specific circumstances, the plight of dying typically pushes us into a corner of defenselessness until we muster the ability to come out swinging. When the Colonel presented in the Emergency Department with respiratory distress, his defenses were weakened, uncertainty heightened and his dire necessity to breathe overtook his decision-making capacity. The important distinction between doing and being right is that we are instructed to "do right" from outside while we intuit "being right" from within.

The same courage that inspires living strong provides strength when it is time to die. Finding dignity amid the uncertainty of death invites us to be both creative and wishful. I can imagine the process of dying becoming the final exam before experiencing the bliss of "School is out!" forever. Does freedom really equate to bliss? A yoga instructor challenged this premise when he set the intention for a particular class with this insight: "Uncertainty is my path to freedom."

Uncertainty is fertile ground for the creative spirit. It casts doubt on any decision-making process of when to go for it or let go. Uncertainty presents the struggle of going to the ED or waiting to be seen in the physician's office. Uncertainty opens any end-of-life conversation with thought-provoking questions. Uncertainty struggles against the fact that something needs to be said about providing more dignity to patients, yet we reluctantly accept this freedom.

Uncertainty is usually scary since most people crave certainty. Too much freedom becomes overwhelming, creating an overabundance of uncertainty and/or irrationality. We may not know exactly what to do when dealing with serious illness, but it is vital to know who we are when confronting such a challenge.

The uncertainty inherent in dying calls every aspect of our being into question. As life is precious, dying feels wrong. How can we be certain we are doing the right thing when facing this possibility? Doubt tends to be heartbreaking rather than empowering. The certainty of "doing" right often directly challenges the certainty of "being" right for many patients in the Emergency Department. Dignity noticeably and quickly evaporates under stress. What I personally wish for is to experience dying with dignity. Yet, sorely missing from a majority of Advance Care Directives are guiding principles that impart and promote dignity. We can only determine the best course of action when dignity has a set standard.

Dying with dignity is highly dependent on both personal responsibility and preparatory work; we need to know what we wish for with a fervent appeal to be cared for with dignity. While discussing the premise of that responsibility, a woman gave me a great example of this dynamic. A friend had given her a book in which she was to write her wishes at random; when it came time to declare her birthday wish, she would have a ready list. She admits she put the book aside and never wrote anything in it. I can similarly see how dignity becomes sidelined along with the assignment to complete an Advance Care Directives that express personal wishes.

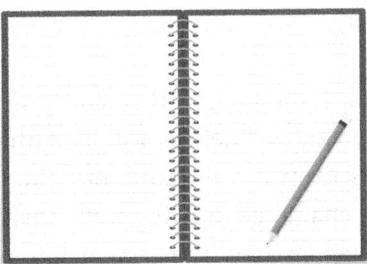

Certain decisions have obvious choices while others create gut-wrenching dilemmas. Good intentions are not enough; we must get this right and it is our personal responsibility. As long as people are capable of making decisions, they continue to claim their dignity? My own Advance Care Directive provides foreknowledge of my decisions at crunch time, when my capacity and communication skills have been diminished by illness or crisis.

Most physicians stand ready to enroll patients in the fight to save their lives. Dignity often implies taking a stand from which we fight for life, longevity and significance. Living longer is invariably dependent upon beating the odds. As self-respect diminishes with age, many people are prone to give more respect to what doctors say than what we hear from within. In general, when people receive the memo that death is imminent, there is no attachment included as to how we might wish for it to occur. Like fate, we take a chance on how we might actually rest in peace.

This touchy, heart-wrenching end of life conversation tends to become avoided. Once patients alert Emergency Medical Services, I find it difficult to throw a wrench into the screeching wheels intent on saving a life. There is great propensity to save life rather than fail. In respecting life at all costs, what becomes of dignity?

Like beauty, dignity is conceived in the eyes of wellness and appears buried within the beast of an illness. Illness is frequently treated in an effort to restore the dignity perceived in being well and feeling worthwhile. When illness overtakes lives and there is no appeal to living, dignity emerges from the perspective of declaring death-defying feats of wellness. Extraordinary measures easily kill the spirit—we know we are dying, but others may refuse to let us go. Instead of peace, we remain in turmoil.

In medical school, I was taught that both illness and wellness are states of mind. In viewing wellness as a state of mind and believing that peace of mind arises from the certainty of being right, it follows that dignity presents as a challenge in dying well. This uphill battle requires a skillset of mind over matter. The responsible course is to consider these issues before our bodies break down. My advance care thinking is not centered on being well, but in appreciating well-being as having adapted to the forces of nature—which includes acquiring the strength to die with dignity.

In a seemingly unhealthy manner, many doctors urge their patients to get well, be right and only die as a last resort. There is little support for a patient to feel right about dying of natural causes that are potentially treatable. Similarly, families will assert the same line of attack: "Are you sure there is nothing more we can do?" I want to stand strong, but in the back of my mind I realize family members prefer the treasure chest of hope is kept wide open. This leads to a potential Pandora's Box of ill-conceived treatments with little regard for the futility of the patient.

The dignity I seek for myself and others at the end of life is not defined with medical terminology, but rather through spiritual awareness. For me, dignity is a spiritual word. Oddly enough, we aspire to dignity in death but spend more time talking about it in medical terms. Typically, Advance Care Directives originate as medical directives, but we should compose them as spiritual initiatives. The current hit-or-miss of dignity being present throughout the process of dying could be traced to the spiritual awareness missing from Advance Care Directives. Wishes, like grace, can be bestowed through Advance Care Directives.

If uncertainty is my path to freedom, then certainty is what will pave my path to dignity. Uncertainty tends to keep all the options on the table; dignity wisely calls on us to select the right option. Uncertainty provides for a change of heart; certainty knows the heart to be absolute. The choice to do "everything" will leave us overwrought with indecision and in indignation.

When appropriate, choosing to die allows a person to leave this life in a less-complicated, more-fulfilled manner. In medical lingo, the "sentinel bleed" or leak from an aneurysm results in a thunderclap headache, a potential a wake-up call. The hope of this book is to clip the aneurysm before life explodes as the worst headache of our uncertainty.

The certainty of being right arises in nature similarly to what occurs at sunrise. At dawn, looking beyond the horizon into the abyss, a groundswell of radiant energy coalesces into a ball of light. This solar plexus, the core of certainty, radiates and reflects the mirror image of our heart's brilliance. The sun intensely shines an inanimate light upon our being.

Teachings of nature, with other divine happenings, shed a similar light on other natural causes that contribute to the certainty of being right. Whether we dig under the surface to find certainty, or allow certainty to simply happen, what speaks to me from the standpoint of dignity is that I am a man who dares to delve into his own heart and espouse self-awareness.

WISH 4:

Self-Awareness

As Benjamin Franklin stated, "... [N]othing is certain but death and taxes." Perhaps the amount of time and consideration we invest in completing income tax forms might also be given to writing Advance Care Directives. The certainty of being right resonates with paying fewer taxes or maximizing tax refunds.

Like many others, I would like to be able to simplify filling out tax forms and Advance Care Directive by using the short form. However, completing the long form, giving thought to itemized deductions and exemptions, raises questions about claiming dependents, earned dividends and interest, bad debts, assets and financial security. In addition, completing the long form may ease the potential pain and suffering of what is paid in the end.

Taking conscious stock of our lives assists in identifying our inherent resources. When confronted with serious illness, the courage of certainty lies largely in knowing ourselves and our ability to draw directly from that awareness. The certainty of being right, particularly at the end of life, begins with painting broad strokes of awareness on three specific aspects of dignity:

- Personal responsibility
- Quality of life
- Highest realization of self

Dying rarely makes sense for any of us who attempt to gain the most from living. Any self-awareness of dying would rarely feel right or provide for certainty. Yet, certainty allows for dignity to be inclusive in both living and dying. Certainty is demonstrated through personal responsibility.

After suffering with pancreatic cancer for six months, a patient finally, reluctantly agreed to hospice care only two days prior to his death.

While his wife had nursed both parents and a sister with cancer through their illnesses and eventual deaths, she appeared taken aback, breaking down emotionally, when informed that her husband was near death. When he died, she inquired where his body would be taken. It was now my turn to be taken aback by the apparent lack of funeral preparations.

If certainty arises from taking personal responsibility, suffering is closely linked to procrastination. If my life has value, so does my time here on earth. Generally, we are responsible for intentions and articles we value. Claiming responsibility for our own deaths seems to some to be treasonous. We are certain we will die, but having a responsible plan for death may be viewed as potentially betraying our lives. When physician initiate end-of-life discussions and encourage patients to put together a responsible plan while dying, patients generally react with anxiety: "What are you telling me, Doctor? What's wrong with me?"

Most physicians realize that more attention needs to be given to discussions of Advance Care Directives, but the talk is framed in abstract wishes rather than concrete responsibilities. The means by which the heart could be resuscitated s discussed when efforts would be better directed toward reconciling what may be futile. Where do we draw the line in receiving life-saving measures? And where does our responsibility lie in communicating these intentions?

Typically, people choose to not think about their own deaths. Denial is an effective coping mechanism. In support of people who smoke or drink while sabotaging their health, the certainty of being right claims, "I have to die of something." The certainty of being right collapses on the idea that death comes when the heart stops. However, acknowledging that we may die of something long before the heart stops makes me wonder if there is more or less personal responsibility hidden in the "something" that suggests dignity. If we acknowledge taking responsibility in perpetrating an illness, would that skew or align with our dignity?

There is relatively little mystery as to why people die. Leading causes are heart disease and cancer followed by COPD, stroke, accident and infection. Many people claim they do not fear death, but could they immediately declare their cause of death? Wishful thinking sets up the preference to die in our sleep with our heads buried under the covers.

When called upon to actually confront death, few have considered how they might expire gracefully. My answer to the Final Jeopardy question in the scheme of life is: "What is 'die from infection'?" From my perspective, these are the quintessential people who die in their sleep.

There are natural causes of death and natural concerns about hastening death. There are natural ways to induce sleep or we can take sleeping pills. Certainty and dignity begin to take shape from personal preferences depending upon what feels right and permits the mind to rest. Primarily, the practice of medicine addresses illness that disrupts wellness. The extraordinary contradiction is that healthcare measures extend our lives unnaturally and sleeping pills may result in more of a hangover than restful sleep.

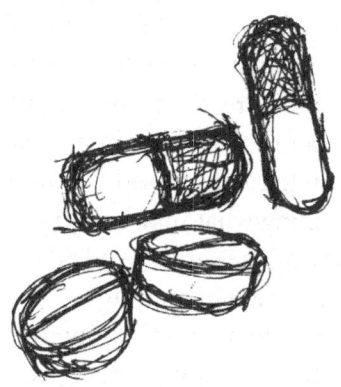

As expectant mothers choose natural childbirth with bravery and commendation, people who choose natural death appear cowardly and are oddly condemned. There are double standards in regard to life and death, wellness and illness. Dignity applies one personal standard that is upheld throughout life and death situations.

Emergency Medicine physicians are trained to plan for the worst-case scenario, addressing it dutifully and responsibly. Intellectually, people realize everyone dies sooner or later. Individuals fail to take responsibility for the loss of their dignity and quality of life when preparations are put off. Obviously, the best care is sought in a crisis situation. Is just making the best of a bad situation good enough? Why not plan for something better? Generally, personal responsibility calls people to determine their own quality of life rather than to take it for granted.

Most of us perceive quality of life as enjoying the comforts of life while free of worry. Some people wait until retirement, or the end of life to expand their time with friends and family. Unfortunately, we tend to equate quality of life with quantity of time. We do everything possible to extend our lives, as if the quantity of years guarantees a quality of life.

If a person is unsure about what deems "quality" of life in the present moment, will that individual be able to recognize when quality of life ends? Quality of life is important, and for selfish reasons. When quality of life ends, I give myself permission to die of natural causes. Quality of life is foremost to any promise of days or years I might potentially live. Healthcare professionals emphasize staying alive, along with encouraging a patient to get well quickly, to get back to a "normal life."

In lieu of doing everything right when quality of life wanes, I wish to impose a treaty and reprieve from further testing and treatments that prolong my life. Each individual defines what quality of life is acceptable, but that definition is never clearly spelled out in Advance Care Directives. The practice of medicine focuses on saving lives and allows patients to justify their quality of life after being saved. Life has an inherent quality to it, like dignity, but defining what it means to an individual seems elusive.

We need to take steps to prioritize what is important in life. Generally, the alcoholic who stumbles into the ED treats relationships as secondary to drinking, while the sedentary person ignores the body's need to be active. Sometimes we choose our quality of life and sometimes the deck is stacked against us. At what point does quality of life decline to an unacceptable level?

Personally, I deem the quality of my life will end when I can no longer live semi-independently. For me, quality of life is perceived in terms of personal freedom, self-reliance and free thought. Living with a disabling illness or injury could be more than I wish to endure. I have no intention of exercising valiant efforts to save my life if I become physically or mentally incapacitated. While I would be willing to accept semi-independence, total dependency is not an option. Empathy allows me to potentially extend this same type of respect to others. However, others first must know, declare and document the stipulations that define and encompass their quality of life.

A physician assistant I work with related that his stepmother experienced a head bleed, resulting in both significant mental and physical impairment. Having become very childlike in her affect, she was no longer the woman his father married. Her quality of life was reduced to requiring total care. Both the PA and I agreed that were we in her shoes, we would have preferred to die much sooner than later. However, without the benefit of an Advance Care Directive listing her wishes, it is presumed she wants all necessary care to sustain her life. When we lack the ability to independently determine quality of life, dignity becomes lost in supposition.

Most living wills lack true clarity and specifics, stating: "If quality of life ends, I no longer want procedures A, B, or C implemented." In a moment of crisis, some patients attempt to disavow their own living wills for the chance to continue breathing. We can easily be coerced into being placed on a ventilator while struggling to breathe or agreeing to a feeding tube when unable to eat. With the devolution that occurs in end-stage disease like COPD or ALS (Amyotrophic lateral sclerosis, also known as Lou Gehrig's disease), quality of life usually becomes questionable when we can no longer say, "At least I still have my health."

Dignity and quality of life become secondary priorities to anyone struggling to breathe. Similarly, the same challenge with panic and suffocation presents while alleviating pain and suffering. This is my job in a nutshell. As soon as I hear patients yelping while entering the Emergency Department, I jump to stomp out all pain and suffering. While in that vice grip of suffering, patients typically welcome any and all interventions to alleviate the pain. "Just make it stop hurting," they plead —*never mind my dignity.*

I usually need to ask several questions in order to understand the reason for a patient's pain. Patients often find this insufferable while I call it my job. When I get a grip on what is triggering their pain, they receive appropriate pain medication. After several repeat visits, patients often tend to demand more certainty than medications to manage their pain. This watershed moment begins to separate the science of medicine from the art of medicine. The art of medicine draws upon self-awareness in distinguishing suffering from pain.

I met a remarkable young man suffering from depression and anxiety. Rather than medication affecting his cure, his mindset affected a cure. He surfed through a sundry of antidepressants that did more to suppress his erections, enhancing his performance anxiety. When he decided his drug of choice was sex, he gave up all medication and learned to catapult his affliction into something more potent and life affirming. His plan of action became self-prescribed. Rarely do I see people escape the oppressive chains of chronic illness. His motivation came from a "can-do" attitude rather than being trapped by some doctor "do-little" circumspection.

The certainty of being treated right originates directly from the core of the person I am treating. When patients wear their intentions on their sleeves rather than hidden up their sleeves, I am better able to discern whether I am treating a person or a patient. When I walk into a room and am greeted by, "Hey Doc, I'm suffering over here," I know I am attending to a patient. By definition, being patient means "to suffer." Even as this patient suffers, self-awareness mandates that suffering may not be necessary. The person becomes in touch with the Zen axiom: *Pain is inevitable, suffering is optional.*

The certainty of being right upfront equates to the self-perception of being man or mouse—human or guinea pig —person or patient. I am often impressed when a perceived "person" presents with significant pain or disease, yet appears devoid of suffering; they seem to see the glass is half full rather than half empty. The conversation begins from the fluid consciousness of that person. Basically, I view patients as being immunocompetent or immunocompromised—possessing either the ability to fight disease without suffering, or the inability to fight disease due to their suffering. Experiencing pain or illness is inevitable throughout life. Having the ability to allay suffering seems optimal.

While many people prefer being treated as a "person," most patients become caught up in their suffering. Typically, these individuals opt for unnecessary tests and procedures or often prefer I take action rather than discuss what may make good sense not to do. Because it seems "everyone else" generally gets an X-ray translates into my not taking the patient seriously or not knowing what I am doing. Patients will often set themselves up for being gullible. I remember a woman with abdominal pain who was waiting to be seen in the ED. She allowed a cervical collar to be placed around her neck that was intended for another patient. Was this woman suffering so much that she would gladly accept anything?

Many patients who appear to be clueless to the effects of stress on their bodies, believing the body is immune to such emotional strain. They can quickly sense the stress of pain, but lack awareness that stress adds to the pain. When the body hurts, suffering undermines quality of life. I become aware of suffering after donning a patient gown. I notice an immediate breeze of vulnerability. At times, suffering makes patients feel taken for granted; this feeling is manifested through their unmet expectations. By the same token, patients who suffer seem to expect care to be readily available without acknowledgment or thanks. The certainty of being right might invite less suffering.

While the highest realization of self does occur through suffering, I perceive dignity evolving from the Buddhists' belief that enlightenment is the end of suffering. In doing the right thing, the shell of dignity appears as being upright and doing things right; yet, I question whether this actually feels right following enlightenment. Personal enlightenment suggests habits are preferred over facts and experience trumps science. An example of this is that some people experience cigarette smoking as calming despite its cancer risk. Who am I to know the mind of another? Yet, yet who are we not to seek enlightenment through our own divine intelligence?

While explaining the medical reasons why someone is near death, the underlying, heartbreaking question is, "Why do I have to die?" Without the answer to this existential question, certainty is apt to be displaced. When dignity escapes self-awareness, the mind creates a free-for-all of anarchy, conflict and indignation. Having witnessed many people in the throes of end-of-life decisions, I can attest to the overwhelming difficulties that emerge from dying without adequate preparation, self-awareness and resolution.

We need to look clearly at the inevitability of death as part of our voyage in life. At some point, the bow of our personal Titanic is going to ram an iceberg. Typically, one of three scenarios plays out. Some people are unwittingly thrown from the bow in the sheer terror of sudden death. Others may initiate a call to 911 and rush to the lifeboat hoping to be saved. Still others may feel right in accepting their fates and take seats with the orchestra playing "Nearer, My God, to Thee."

The certainty of dying with dignity is best achieved through introspection, self-awareness and self-direction. Advance Care Directives are contingency plans for when things go awry. Typically, these plans begin with listening to the doctor. My personal contingency plan is to reconcile my thoughts and emotions prior to having these conversations. I listened intently to a recent radio interview featuring an end-of-life counselor. At the end of the program, the host probed the counselor for her own end-of-life plan. I turned up the volume.

"Oh, I'm sure my children will know what to do." She had chosen her daughter, a midwife, to be her medical power of attorney. Her son would be there to help. Nothing had been clearly delineated, no contingency plan outlined; I was surprised this counselor's command seemed designed to pass the buck. The show motivated me to rewrite my original manuscript to demonstrate how to create a plan of action that would outline how life is to end, while simultaneously maintaining command of dignity.

Wishes To Die For is a road map for that journey to self-awareness. In distinguishing my own person journey, I realize I am a spiritual being living a human existence. Consequently, I bring my spirituality into my profession when emotionally connecting with patients. Through an appreciation of this connection, I tend to suffer when patients suffer. I also realize that we are subject to two deaths at the end of life: physical death and spiritual death. What becomes challenging is sustaining physical life when the spirit seems to have passed. These situations call for self-restraint from the unrealistic expectations of the healthcare system.

WISH 5:

Self-restraint Regarding Healthcare

The great poet Rumi ascribes, "I should be suspicious of what I want." Like many others, as I become older I look forward to Medicare paying for healthcare expenses. Being enrolled in Medicare makes healthcare available, yet access to healthcare does not ensure good health. Eating an apple a day keeps the doctor away, but once people can afford to get sick by having healthcare, I witness people choosing to see the doctor rather than consuming the healthy option of an organic apple.

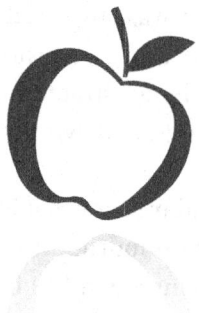

The certainty of being right careens into the certainty of being taken for a ride when becoming ill. I stand in suspicion of people who believe they are treated well as I prescribe a multitude of medication and tests that conflict with my sense of living well. Are people becoming more realized as patients and less recognized as people?

Statistically, the older we become, the more likely it is for us to become ill and be hospitalized. Younger patients are more likely to take risks with their heath, making boastful claims of not having seen a doctor in many years. I recently treated a 32-year-old man who had been diagnosed with a hole in his heart septum. Once again he had passed out during sex. He did not have insurance and could not afford medication. However, he seemed content in not taking medication and had been compensating fairly well physically. His comfort level with risk rather than medication suggested something to me about dignity. The ability to take risk along with the certainty of being right may actually be a useful tool in self-restraint.

If what you don't know won't hurt you, then what you do know may hurt when certain medical treatments or lifestyle changes become necessary. Generally, younger people tend to be cavalier and offhanded with what they believe they know. They may know that excess sun exposure, sugar intake, and smoking are unhealthy, but frequently prefer not to discontinue these behaviors. Are medical tests necessary to promote and maintain being health conscious? Do we need to know our specific cholesterol level before choosing low-cholesterol foods? Is sun protection a forethought or an afterthought to skin cancer? I believe living life to the fullest allows us to engage in disease prevention behavior balanced with middle-of-the-road indulgence.

For some elderly patients, the go-to plan of Advance Care Directives is to worry themselves sick. They already tend to be fearful of dying and easily become overly focused or fixated on heart attacks and strokes, prompting checking their blood pressures incessantly. Higher readings occur as a consequence.

People often repeat the cliché that it is *better to be safe than sorry*. This one phrase greatly extends the line of patients waiting to be seen in the Emergency Department. However, I am not convinced that playing it safe actually supports certainty. The more I dwell on dignity, the stronger I advocate for certainty over worry. By playing it safe, do we attract what we fear? Fear results in anxiety and overthinking, working against reasonable judgment and self-restraint.

Historically, Advance Care Directives have been written from the perspective of attempting to prolong life. I view these documents as catalysts to creating destiny. It is not the occurrence of the stroke or cancer that shapes my future, but how I choose to react to illness. The deeper we plunge, falling head over heels into the healthcare system, the more difficult it becomes to maintain self-restraint. While I am certain that a majority of patients have preconceived notions of when enough is enough, most rarely decline the extended warranty offered through comprehensive healthcare. When is it better to be safe in a nursing home than sorry to have ended up there? I believe we need to be suspicious of what we want long before wishing to receive any treatment.

Most Advance Care Directives are formulated to play it safe and are often equated with preservation. I preface safety and preservation with dignity. I view implementing an Advance Care Directive as going out on a limb that may eventually break. The so-called "safety net" easily traps us in a web of complacency. Decisions regarding what we do and do not treat are normally left to healthcare professionals who assume authority. I suggest maintaining personal authority in these matters.

As an educator, a physician is capable of explaining disease processes and answering questions about potential complications. However, a physician need never be the final word in deciding which options are right for the patient. The doctor can offer further testing and treatment, but cannot be 100 percent certain of providing the absolute right treatment. Patients are encouraged to understand their roles in making treatment decisions personalized.

Doubts that surround death and dying present an opportunity to raise consciousness. Advance Care Directives become homework assignments for adults. Similarly to a child's approach to homework, adults might adopt coping strategies utilized when avoiding death and dying, i.e. denial, bargaining, anger, depression and acceptance. Setting aside and avoiding these life and death homework assignments leads to chaos, confusion and contention among family, friends, caregivers and professionals involved in end-of-life care.

There is usually no self-restraint in living life to the fullest when dealing with terminal illness. What distinguishes homework from classwork is when a child works independently. When children are left to their own devices, fear of failure runs rampant, permits an individual to dawdle in denial. Unlike Elisabeth Kübler-Ross, who was sensitive to how individuals cope with each stage of dying at their own pace, my mother advocates, "Don't put off until tomorrow what can be done today." Procrastination is averted by creating Advance Care Directives, and that lead to certainty over helplessness by discovering what someone is able to do on their my own.

I remember Dr. Reider from my residency training stating, "What you don't do will come back to haunt you," but many other people chose to believe, "What you don't know won't hurt you." Unfortunately, that can come back to haunt them. Death is not necessarily frightening. It is not knowing the hurt, indignation and shackles that might precede death. Fear tightens the screws that make it more difficult to die, particularly when having a hand in it. Loosening the screw in order to let go, I remember my father's wisdom: "Don't screw it in so tight; that only makes it harder to get out."

When we no longer feel right in life, we risk becoming caught in a bind. Holding on to the right to life while no longer feeling right creates a pickle. I recall a sweet elderly woman approaching the nurse's station and saying, "I'm in pee-col." The innocence and casualness in her tone while recognizing the walls were closing in made me giggle. She was not up against a life or death situation; however, it was in her best interest to stay in the hospital where she could receive the care she needed despite its potential antiseptic brine.

Life happens while we are busy getting into pickles. Having Advance Care Directives in place offers respite from these inevitable situations. As dying patients recognize they are becoming weaker, it may be time to consider discontinuing medication or treatment designed to prolong life. Patients may recognize they are relying on physicians and medications to feel right about dying, but real certainty is self-adjudicated.

Having an established relationship with doctors becomes an open invitation for individuals to manage their overall health. This relationship becomes solidified when medications are prescribed and need to be refilled. Physicians need to be aware of and to question when medications begin to sabotage health, contributing to the delinquency of patients. Medication lists give me some idea of how dignity has been supplanted when health becomes over-supplemented.

Medications can be perceived as citations to health. Patients or family members begin to question, "Are these medications all necessary?" These questions reflect self-examination on the patient's part. There are always choices in deferring on medication, particularly as death draws near or when supporting natural death. Few doctors are going to tell patients not to take medication.

While I remain committed to patients maximizing their health, I prefer to engage patients in the certainty of feeling right regarding healthcare decisions. Generally, this is a conversation I would prefer pursuing further, but my ability to do so is constrained by time allotted in the ED. As there are two sides to every conversation, there are two sides to my opinion as well—both personal and professional. Patients rarely compare the treatment plan I offer against inquiring what I might do personally.

The two primary processes in physician-patient interaction consist of diagnosis and doing. The physician provides the diagnosis, but too often patients ultimately fail to take responsibility for the doing, failing to fill their prescriptions, return to doctors for follow-up visits or complete recommended outpatient testing. Doctors cannot do everything. There are certain questions about end-of-life care that can only be answered from within the person. This is where dignity needs to become part of the dialogue that leads to patient empowerment. *Do or die* should be balanced with not doing and still dying.

For some, dignity implies thorough investigation that ensures nothing is missed. For others, dignity involves self-restraint and selecting only what is deemed necessary to create certainty. Whichever side a patient deems right is usually the starting point regarding healthcare decisions. Generally, I suggest minimal testing to expedite care and lessen the prospects of tests that may result in false positives. Most patients initially concur with this plan, but some ask for more testing, thinking this may lead to certainty. Even when patients are certain an injured limb is not broken, few are willing to forgo an X-ray. To avoid creating contention, I order the unnecessary X-ray that remains important to them.

Negating what seems to be the "right thing" creates anxiety. Even when death is certain, the right thing to do seems to prevent people from dying. Most Advance Care Directives advocate life support before calling it quits. The consciousness impacting end-of-life decisions includes family member attitudes, healthcare workers' opinions, underlying fear and personal faith. Encouraging increased consciousness of self-restraint, provide for more peaceful settlements and transitions.

Healthcare is a bureaucracy, a system built upon specialized functions that adhere to orders and protocols. The individual's power is left to the mercy of the system. A dying patient's desire for certainty and affirmation becomes shrouded and suppressed in the shuffle of paperwork, healthcare rules and regulations. There are two battles to be waged at the end of life. The first occurs in fighting an illness; the second is the bureaucracy that prolongs life. Even when patients come to terms with their impending deaths, discharge orders that permit them to die could take months or years to be processed and signed.

The saying, "You can't fight city hall" is reminiscent of the futility of waging war against bureaucracy. The best course of action in any fight is to enlist a higher power. The heart-center is an individual's higher power and the absolute decision-maker regarding the appropriate time to die.

WISH 6:

Self-Deference to the Heart-Center

A spunky 70-year-old woman with a sharp wit and friendly disposition—was visiting from California and presented with a three-week history of fever and abdominal pain. She had recently received treatment for a lingering *H. Pylori* infection in her stomach. My evaluation in the Emergency Department revealed metastatic liver disease, with the primary cancer originating in her colon. Intuitively, she had a hunch she might have cancer and was prepared for this diagnosis. She accepted that her endpoint was to die of cancer, but didn't seem to have given much thought to how she might proceed with this information.

As she lay smiling in the ED, she informed her family that she was at peace with the diagnosis. Her attitude clearly communicated, "Let your heart not be troubled," embracing the diagnosis with an unusual eagerness to move on with the process. The next steps would include admitting her to the hospital, pursuing additional tests and then discussing treatment options. But if someone is ready to die and presumably prefers to die at home, why be admitted? Why follow the protocol?

In retrospect, I wish I had discussed distinguishing the prospect of care in regards to her wishes and not what would be considered standard care. Two weeks later she returned to the ED with a bowel obstruction following "the process"—surgery to remove her colon.

What she seemed to wish for and what she was put through were contradictory. Her strengths were her pleasant demeanor and accommodating personality. She embraced the healthcare system as comprised of wonderful people, but negated her spirited passion that embraced death. If she was ready to die with the certainty of being right, she had come to the wrong place and was being "treated" to death. In being overly accommodating, it seemed she was getting killed in the process.

I hoped to learn much from this patient's journey; particularly, how she cultivated this readiness to die. While her personal conviction was admirable, I was perplexed and upset that she did not have a plan to avoid being roped into prolonging her life. She was ready to die and did not know how to determine her course. The situation prompted me to delve deeper into my own aspirations regarding dying. What treatments would I refuse? My former Advance Care Directive simply selected various means of life support. This was just skimming the surface; so I set about creating a more comprehensive Advance Care Directive.

Most of us have difficulty forecasting how we will react to life-threatening situations—when we come face-to-face with dying. We wish for unlimited knowledge and awareness, divine intervention or certainty. Where is God in this moment?

Intellectually, people believe the right thing to do is to remain in the hospital, urgently completing any and all available testing procedures. Meditation provides calm and creates a quiet place where we can listen to our hearts, free from the distractions of fear.

If possible, with a little time, the right thing for me would be to go home and sleep on it; take the time to *pause, center and shift*. This concept was foundational to the seminar titled, "Initiation into the Heart Center" conducted by H. Brugh Joy, MD. A pulmonologist and mystic, Dr. Joy was a great aficionado of the heart-center. The heat radiating from the space between the lungs constantly intrigued him. The heart-space, with its molten bed of effusive and magnetic energy, challenged him to dig deeper into its mysteries.

In the awareness that everything happens for a reason, Brugh insisted, "the heart deletes the need to understand." Certainty is rarely available in highly perplexing situations. During any illness a lapse of certainty will occur and patients long for a supportive connection to a higher power. The mindful directive to "follow your heart," traversing thinking to and through the heart, often provides a sense of direction. When focused on the mind to figure things out, we more likely become stuck in procrastination instead of bowing to the heart's intuition.

The heart declares the reason we live and die through the certainty of divine providence.

Spiritual discipline occurs through quieting the mind and listening to the heart. For this insight and benefit, in addition to practicing medicine, I practice yoga. The connection bridging these two disciplines occurs through the heart-space. The heart-center awakens an alternative state of consciousness in caring for others as I care for myself. Becoming present to the mind-body connection occurs in yoga. Deepening into my core is not only valuable to my life, but is a gift that is meant to be both applied to the end of my life and shared with others.

While exploring the heart-center, I envision my soul. The mystery of the soul tends to remain two-fold: where it is located and what it reveals. With its pervasive and elusive quality, the soul connects our humanity with divinity. As experiences lift my heart and enlighten my mind, I feel my soul rejoice. Therefore, it is not a stretch to appreciate the soul as the sac surrounding my heart. As a crucible, my heart unites my existence to the universe. As I incorporate what is universal into that which is personal, all life is eternal and my soul honors both my presence on the earth and my presence beyond the earth. Given the two aspects of the soul, one side tells me, "In God we trust" while the flip side contracts with the devil to die.

A negative change in health status presents the opportunity to *pause, center and shift* from illness being solely fact-based to becoming a faith-based intention arising from the soul. The certainty of healing and not healing is understood through the soul. Through the practice of yoga, I continually defer to my heart-space as I prayerfully place my hands upon my chest for assurance. Joy eloquently described the resources of the heart-center as "attributes." The mystery of the heart is realized through these attributes that offer solace to the mystery of life.

With hands overlying his heart, Brugh explored and espoused four gifts that arise from the heart: *compassion, innate harmony, healing presence and unconditional love.* Comingling these attributes upon the stages of grief from the work of Elisabeth Kübler-Ross created a foundation and example for my own Advance Care Directive: denial and anger overcome by *compassion*—bargaining negotiated through *innate harmony*—depression submersed into the heart's *healing presence*—and acceptance attained through *unconditional love.*

Decision-making capacity is constrained by the mind, but becomes expansive while exploring these attributes of the heart. The mind is discerning, judgmental and exclusive of death; the heart is directive, intuitive, and inclusive of death. Through the practice of yoga, I am reminded that as we ground our feet, we push down to ascend—plant to grow—and root to rise—giving certainty to our stance and resolve.

Using these distinctions, Advance Care Directives originate best from the heart, not from the mind. The guide to *pause, center and shift* is an opportunity to lay the foundation before beginning any course of action. Similar variations of this cautious theme include stop, look and listen; stop, drop and roll; eat, pray, love; DOWN…SET…HIKE! This football analogy creates a type of mission statement for Advance Care Directives: The goal of spiking the ball at the end of life comes with the intention to nail it, get it right and win.

In life, death remains an unavoidable part of the end game. The football "receiver" generally proceeds to the end zone with intention and zeal, evading the least amount of pain, injury and interference. Closer to the end zone, the defensive efforts of well-intentioned healthcare providers and caregivers often intensify and prevent the person from dying. It is more likely that the person will be tackled rather than make it gracefully into the end zone. Buried beneath the defensive players, one may have little space to move and much less ability to breathe. When the virtual referee dismantles the pileup of players, I perceive dignity remaining in the person at the bottom of the pack who maintains possession of the ball.

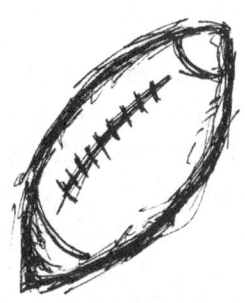

In regulation play, the clock stops when the touchdown is complete. However, time is still allotted for kicking the extra point. Adopting a similar rule to advance care planning, patients might consider strategies for effectively reaching their declared end points and then coming to terms with proper end-of-life care. Naturally, the dynamic and intensity of the game switches as special teams (hospice) descend on the field to assist the kicker (patient). Advance Care Directive often address interventions that are to be withheld from patients than rather medical options that allow patients to rest in peace. Advance care planning has to include introspection and discussion regarding appropriate care measures that follow the final "touchdown."

The playbook of an Advance Care Directive has to include game plans and strategies for how best to handle difficult situations rationally and intuitively. Certain plays will be completed as expected while others result in the ball being fumbled and people scrambling for control of it. Ideally, the ball remains on your side of the field with thoughtful consideration being given to many fourth-down situations that call for punting, throwing caution to the wind or running the clock out. The analogy of four downs being given to those who have possession of the ball can be applied to people addressing their Advance Care Directives in four stages:

1. Commencement of Advance Care Directives
2. Preamble of Advance Care Directives
3. Enactment of Advance Care Directives
4. Deliverance through Advance Care Directives

The appeal of this book is a personal goal to explore concepts, create doctrine and possibly propose legislation that will guide and empower others to expand their living wills into conscientious Advance Care Directives, aligning personal preferences with a Universal Healthcare Directive. With an outline comprised of the commencement, preamble, enactment and deliverance regarding Advance Care Directives, we might further explore the standpoint of dignity in both stages of living and dying. Dignity flows freely when the heart is in the game. By incorporating attributes of the heart into the process of creating Advance Care Directives, we commence along the journey that leads to the certainty of being right.

PART II

...

*Commencement Of
Advance Care Directives*

WISH 7:

Pre-Counsel and Guidance

I was raised to be a responsible adult. My parents taught me obedience, discipline, duty, achievement and respect. Beyond caring about my sensitivities or their sacrifices, the implied directive was for me to attain a place in Heaven. Naturally, there were differences of opinion along the way and even questions about the existence of Heaven. Nevertheless, these obstacles never excused me from being morally responsible and living with dignity. My parents' wishes, along with Led Zeppelin's lyrics instilled the sense of buying the "stairway" to Heaven.

Unconscious thoughts about Advance Care Directives arose while kneeling with my kid-siblings in a narrow hallway and facing a crucifix adorned with a basket-weaved palm leave hanging on the wall. Within arm's reach was a crucible of holy water for blessing ourselves with the sign of the cross. Above us was an attic fan drawing both air and our messages to Heaven. Hands folded in prayer, we recited our inaugural advance care petition:

> *Now I lay me down to sleep,*
> *I pray the Lord my soul to keep.*
> *If I should die before I wake,*
> *I pray the Lord my soul to take.*

Potential substitutes for the final line of this familiar bedtime prayer include:

> *. . . Then it be my fate.*
> *. . . Teach me the path of love (dignity) to take.*

Through a profession in Emergency Medicine, I also contemplate:

> *. . . Call 911 to resuscitate.*

. . . I pray Do Not Resuscitate.
. . . I pray my Advance Care Directive is up-to-date.

At a young age, we learn that all people eventually die and that dying in our sleep is the best hope for a peaceful death. However, questions about what pleases the Lord while confronting treatment options for terminal illness might prevent me from sleeping at night. Teach me the path of dignity to take suggests devising a straightforward path paved with good intentions and clear expectations. My game plan at the end of life strives to Advance to Go with a "get out of jail free" card and collect certainty before amassing a $200,000 hospital bill.

Contemplating death at a relatively young age seems morbid, but it can prove to be both educational and instructional. Given the emotional deluge that occurs at the end of life, it is wise to consider how we prime the pump before the deluge of emotions start overflowing. Do we realize having a hand in the up-and-down energy expended?

At the age of six, I vaguely remember my grandmother dying of liver cancer. With her jaundiced, coarse skin, my first impression of dying was that of a person shriveled into the unhallowed shell of a pumpkin. It reminded me of how Cinderella had been warned to leave the ball before midnight or her carriage would turn back into a pumpkin. Had Grandma stayed too long at the ball?

Traditional Halloween celebrations expose children to frightening scenes: morbid displays of tombstones in cemeteries, haunted houses with decaying bodies and moaning ghosts rattling oppressive chains. These images still give me the heebie-jeebies. Pregnant zombies, devils, witches, trauma victims, patients with catheters and characters from *One Flew Over the Cuckoo's Nest* are simply another night in the Emergency Department. I appreciate this setting as being the mortuary of our mortality.

Raised Catholic, my earliest concept of death and dying was centered around three days: the mock-horrors of Halloween (All Hallows' Eve), the glory of All Saints' Day, and the cautionary mention of All Souls' Day. We honored saints for the selfless struggles they endured for the greater good. They offered up martyrdom as an example of living with purpose and dignity. For those who were less than faithful, All Souls' Day acknowledged the poor souls sent to purgatory. These souls were required to serve penance, waiting for sufficient prayers of others to procure each of them a place in heaven.

My end-of-life plan as a young child was to avoid becoming a poor soul sent to detention. Simultaneously, I stockpiled prayers for poor souls and attempted to avoid the near occasion of sin. I worried about whether people would pray for me after I was gone. My parents stressed the importance of being good while continuing to remind me of my shortcomings; certainly, I was destined for purgatory. Being ambitious, disciplined and sensitive to helping others and myself, a career in medicine seemed to serve my ideal of saving poor souls and winning favor from God. This seed was planted, sprouted and began to grow when I was accepted into the pre-med program at Saint Louis University.

During the summer prior to entering college I was inducted into the halls of purgatory while training to become a certified nurse assistant. Armed with the dream of helping poor souls, I obtained employment in the orthopedic section at a nearby hospital. The fruits of my labor were realized in bones healing and patients moving beyond their physical setbacks. My heart was completely invested in this entry-level position and my passion grew through receiving affirmation from both patients and staff. Serendipitously, one day I found myself caring for the husband of the nursing director of the hospital's Emergency Department. Two weeks later I was caring for her patients in the ED.

Immediately after college graduation I spent the summer with a friend on the east coast. To finance our road trips, we worked at a nursing home. I became reacquainted with the halls of purgatory, where poor souls with hip fractures are sent when they fail to recover, developing bedsores that add to their misery and penance. While there, I bonded with a young male patient who had sustained traumatic brain injury and was restricted to a wheelchair. Trusting in miracles, I encouraged him to walk each day in the hopes of him leaving this ungodly institution. I was naive and starry-eyed while thinking *if you believe it, you can achieve it.* The summer ended before he had regained the ability to walk.

When I entered medical school at Southern Illinois University, I had a better understanding of why this man with brain trauma would never walk again. However, empathy put me squarely in the middle of his shoes. I worked first to help him, then to help myself. This made me think, "What would I do if I was unable to walk again and was sentenced to an extended-care facility?" After finding my niche in Emergency Medicine at Mercy Medical Center in Saint Louis, I continued to care for poor souls from these types of facilities. Each time I searched for the person buried beneath the devastation of their illness, I questioned whether my care was truly helping them or not.

Being young, robust and healthy, I gave little consideration to the possibility of ever being placed in a long-term care facility. One morning while driving home after work my eyelids were drooping and my head was bobbing. Conceivably, if I was in an accident and suffered brain trauma, I could end up in the earthly purgatory with my adopted buddy. I immediately wrote a living will specifically stating that if I ever incurred severe brain injury, I was not to be brought through the revolving door of the ED. I would be ready for the afterworld.

I did not wish to rely on others' prayers on behalf of my soul. Therefore, I had an attorney incorporate my specific wishes into the standard form of an Advance Care Directive. By completely removing the option of being transported to the ED, I opened the possibility of not implementing other acute care measures to purposefully prolong my life. I checked "no" to every option listed on my Advance Care Directive, believing that if I did not have the intellectual capacity for informed consent, no other intervention was warranted. While my attorney clearly understood these wishes, he was uncertain whether existing law would allow these restrictive wishes to be honored, particularly without being officially diagnosed as having a terminal illness or being in a persistent vegetative state. What about my right to die with self-determination?

I continued treating poor souls while praying for my own, but wondered how I might ensure dying expeditiously. I wanted my say, but have always believed that others need more of a say, particularly when they are deemed incompetent. Never wishing to dismiss the value of an individual patient always challenges the intention of withholding care from this patient. "You go first." "No, you go first," is the kind of hesitation that occurs while commencing this discussion. A shift in the delivery of end-of-life care is needed—one that allows individuals to express their wishes ahead of time instead of simply acquiescing to obligations. The focus of my care is not on deciphering patients' wishes, but on granting reasonable wishes that enrich the end of life while honoring free will.

Before I began practicing medicine, Karen Ann Quinlan was lying in a persistent vegetative state. Much of the impetus to draft Advance Care Directives originally arose from issues regarding her medical care and the ensuing legal and moral considerations. In 1975, she stopped breathing due to a drug overdose that resulted in severe brain damage. After spending several months in a persistent vegetative state, the hospital refused to discontinue life support as had been requested by her parents. With Ms. Quinlan's dignity at stake, a lengthy court battle proceeded and her parents' certainty of being right prevailed. Eventually, the breathing tube was removed. Ms. Quinlan survived another decade by means of a feeding tube until she died of pneumonia. My hunch is that obligatory antibiotics were administered before she was finally allowed to die.

Early on in my practice, Terri Schiavo was another high profile patient in a persistent vegetative state. Ms. Schiavo's predicament involved removal of the feeding tube, the same means by which Karen Ann Quinlan's life was sustained. Her husband's certainty of her wish and right to die was in direct conflict with that of her parents' desire to keep her fed. Battle lines were soon drawn across the country. The issue was debated in the court system and beyond, even the halls of Congress. I am certain that most people would not prefer an Act of Congress to give them permission to die. Government and judicial interference in major life decisions can be averted by documenting specific personal end-of-life wishes well in advance.

Just one year after Ms. Schiavo's death, the former prime mister of Israel, Ariel Sharon, 77, suffered a brain hemorrhage that caused a debilitating stroke. Mr. Sharon was in a persistent vegetative state that required ventilator support to sustain his life. In the past and in consultation with neurosurgery, I would rarely place this type of dire patient on life support for fear they would be kept alive indefinitely. At present, this would be considered medical negligence. I was intrigued by Prime Minister Sharon's situation, wondering just how long the life of a renowned dignitary would be prolonged. The answer finally came when he died eight years later.

These recurring events spark concern about having life prolonged while in a persistent vegetative state (a wakeful unconscious state lasting longer than a few weeks). This is a powerful wake-up call at any age, given the frequency of brain injury. Generally, these perilous situations trigger a *fight or write* response. What is morally appropriate? Being mindful of personal wishes and documenting these in Advance Care Directives lessens the likelihood of anyone being treated as a ward of the state.

When treating an unresponsive terminally ill prison inmate in respiratory distress who lacked having a "get out of jail free" card, both he and I were jointly handcuffed by the system. I had no recourse but to place him on a ventilator. Implementation of Advance Care Directives assists in carefully expressing end-of-life wishes. As a type of "get out of jail free" card, my Advance Care Directive is designed to avert the legal and emotional traps that may potentially undermine my claim to dignity.

Most patients who present to the ED without Advance Care Directives essentially become wards of the state, automatically receiving life-prolonging measures. With the intention to always preserve life, docs become cops in the duty to protect and serve. While strapped onto a gurney and hoisted into the paddy wagon of an ambulance, there is an assumption that the patient has rights. But without a clear directive, those rights default to someone being treated like those who wish everything be done to sustain life. As provided by law, we retain the right to make one call to our medical power of attorney. The hope is that this "savior" will prevent unusual or cruel punishment and free us from becoming virtual pawns in the healthcare system.

Standard operating procedure typically takes precedent during emergency situations. At the scene of an accident, people may commence with the certainty of being all right until paramedics voice doubts, causing them to have second thoughts. Frequently, people agree to abide by the protocol of being strapped to a backboard with the intention of being safe rather than sorry. When I release the straps, do my exam and find that patients appear to be all right, I get pushback from those who feel sheepish. Seemingly, the system worked against their initial certainty of being right. What commences as people playing it safe frequently results in side effects of remorse and humiliation for having been overly cautious.

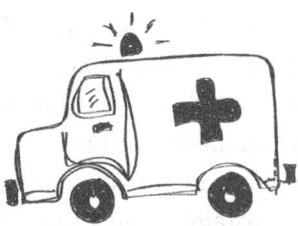

As a rule of law, standard operating procedures do save lives. This is why first responders follow these protocols. However, one size does not fit all. Individuals can become conscientious objectors. In this context, they may prefer taking more direct paths to die, guided by straightforward information. To be talked to straight implies maintaining an even or erect posture of strength that aligns with dignity. The words and wishes that comprise Advance Care Directives become the necessary building blocks for our spines to maintain proper alignment. When all is said and done, the certainty of being right is congruent to having a spine with a supportive document.

WISH 8:

Pre-End-of-Life Plan

Most Advance Care Directives commence when a person is encouraged to complete a pre-printed form in conjunction with other important estate planning documents. A will is created to distribute our assets, decide who may raise children, consider organ donation and determine cremation or burial. All too often these forms are completed with insufficient introspection regarding our specific desires that discern life-sustaining measures in the event of chronic, terminal, disabling disease or injury. These undying situations require forethought, yet are frequently glossed over with consideration only being given to them when the time comes.

After Advance Care Directives are completed, it is easy to become lulled into a false sense of security—*I pray the Lord my soul to take.* Advance Care Directives must be periodically reviewed and revised to keep them current. *Wishes To Die For* assists patients in approaching the end of life constructively, while challenging fear that perpetuates the need to prolong life at any cost. In learning to snowboard, I was instructed not to look directly at trees I wished to avoid hitting. Wherever our eyes go, the body tends to follow. Hence, it becomes imperative to keep our vision focused directly on wishes, not fears.

The assumption that people all have the right to die amid prayers *for the Lord my soul to take* is not in alignment with the perceived moral obligation to save lives. The general consensus of *the Lord my soul to take* arises from an acceptance and agreement that death is imminent. However, herein lays the catch. When two physicians agree that saving a life has become futile, lifesaving measures cease. The concept of two people actually reaching a mutual agreement about this futility may appear to be simple, but caution frequently usurps certainty, as few physicians wish to play God. While I am able to find primary care physicians willing to sign death certificates, locating another physician willing to act as co-conspirator in the death of a patient is extremely difficult, at best.

There is no time like prime time to pray, *actuate* and create Advance Care Directives; but knowing when to *activate* the specifics of the directives is challenging. Most people take considerable efforts to sustain their lives up to a point. However, what remains elusive is this point of no return. When does it become best to cease life-prolonging measures? Are we ever certain? What if there might be a miraculous medical breakthrough right around the corner? Do we wait for this miracle to occur? My point of no return is when illness moves beyond the medical system's capability of allowing me to live semi-independently. The better part of valor is to *actuate* an Advance Care Directive prior to reaching the point of no return and *activate* the directive after crossing that point.

One wonderful aspect of being in the prime of life is feeling physically centered. Viewing life as spanning the length of a 100-yard (year) football field, the fifty-yard line provides the best perspective of the game. Being of sound mind and body at the peak of life, we presumably have the capacity to make rational decisions. The best time to make a rational decision is clearly from the top of a hill rather than from the valley of death. Before going *over the hill*, we have the ability to take in the stirring panoramic view, writing purposeful and profound intentions in Advance Care Directives.

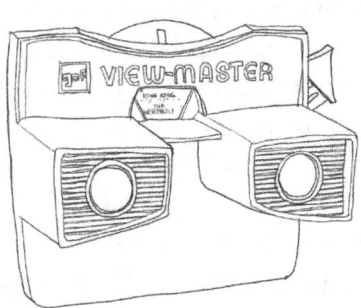

When we make a wish and blow out the candles on our 45th birthday, serious consideration needs to be given to how life might be extinguished through Advance Care Directives. My idea is to create a "deadline" at the prime of life, not waiting until the end of life. The obvious time to take a dignified stand is from a position of strength, celebration and honor. All too often I ask elderly patients to make end-of-life decisions while they prefer to see no evil, hear no evil and speak no evil. This becomes all too confusing, overwhelming, shaming and condemning. Occasionally, I find myself telling patients what to think, while naturally being expected to inform them of their choices and implied decisions to be made. In matters of life and death, I prefer to be objective and have a patient's personal and reasonable wishes expressly documented.

At the middle of life it is possible to read the writing on the wall. At the end of life the print may be too difficult to read. At this point, it generally becomes clear that people have little comprehension of any words that convey prospects of dying. When reading the writing on the wall through premonition or family history, it is important to transcribe this message into a detailed plan of action. For example, how would we handle a stroke? Peace of mind arises from integrity—not simply knowing what we prefer to do, but having the ability to communicate this to others effectively. Integrity speaks of being certain of death, commencing a responsible plan regarding death and dying.

We may attempt to defy aging at all cost, but this need not preclude us from growing old while reaping the benefits of living until a ripe—not spoiled—old age. By midterm, approximately age 45, we have likely declared some certainty about having children. We probably know ourselves as family/relationship-oriented or person/career-oriented; religious or nonreligious; vegetarian or meat eater; excitement seeker or homebody; anti-aging, fitness fanatic or couch potato; having a self-realized or unexamined life. Every individual has the potential to be President of the United States; however, by the age of 45 we likely know whether or not we possess the wherewithal to actually be elected. At this stage in life we begin the process of clearing and paving the path of preference amid self-realization.

For those of us challenged by the idea of growing up or going over the hill, I imagine the thought of dying will cause undue stress. My notion of growing up is finding contentment in life—realizing a profound sense of completeness with little need to prove anything. Prior to my 25th high school reunion, a questionnaire was mailed to the graduation class in order to gather updates on fellow classmates. This opportunity caused me to reflect on what made my life interesting and what still remained on my bucket list. What intrigued me most was the idea of no longer needing to accomplish anything—my life could be complete. As my brother often joked, "Have not, want not!"

My Advance Care Directive is to be implemented when I "have not" quality of life and I "want not" to live. However, there will likely be no shortage of people offering me exactly what I do not want. In fact, there are Good Samaritan laws to protect people who provide reasonable assistance to those in peril, injured or ill, perhaps forcing them to live with a "have not" quality of life. My Advance Care Directive insists Good Samaritans respect my wishes and not attempt to dissuade me from the "want not" of my end-of-life journey. I understand that my right to die might easily be perceived as immoral and be overruled by the extreme moral consciousness that proclaims it is never right to die. This type of righteousness infringes on my certainty of being right.

It is best to come to terms with death before it comes to terms with us. Coming to terms with "growing up" is an alert to draft a term paper on dying with dignity that is due by age 45. Moreover, I strongly recommend that Advance Care Directives be reviewed and revised at each successive mid-decade birthday. Perceptions change as life unfolds and ailments occur; perhaps at 55. 65, 75, etc. These milestones signal a middle ground from where to strengthen the foundation that supports ongoing life-and-death decisions. They also provide an invaluable opportunity to *pause, center and shift* in order to reflect upon being in the midst of our lives, as well as future steps and possible entitlements.

At the age of 45 we most likely have an appreciation of what it means to "pay it forward" regarding retirement entitlements. At 75, entitlements are simply guaranteed. Being middle-aged, I believe in limiting entitlements. However, my mother frets over any limits to hers. When entitlements are guaranteed, we are not necessarily expected to act in a responsible manner. At 45 we hope to know best when to provide a handout and when to pull the plug on hopeless situations. In living longer there are more unjust aspects to illness and disability that occur. There is a prevailing belief that we deserve more out of life.

Dignity garners certainty in how and when to refuse entitlements. The first half of life focuses on success and future entitlements, while the second half of life is focused on upsets and transitions. Certainty provides individuals the knowledge to better understand which boxes to check on Advance Care Directives. Chronic pain and ailments tend to take the focus off the middle ground of the heart-space as patients can easily become self-centered. It is wise to formulate exactly what dignity might afford us before receiving disability services.

When a colleague of mine was anticipating her first child, she and her husband created a series of bylaws and rules as to how they would raise their daughter. Would her daughter receive a new car on her 16th birthday? Would she be allowed to have a dog? In essence, they were adopting a strategy of rationality before the emotional impact of their little girl would soften their stance as parents. I laughed initially, but this idea spoke to me about pre-planning entitlements. Hopefully, at the successive ages of 55 and 65 we will have more accomplishments than needs for entitlements. Perhaps this will translate into more items being checked off bucket lists than *yes* boxes checked on living wills.

What items remain on a personal bucket list? Midlife is a good time to prioritize expectations and determine a timeline for their completion. It seems rational that the more goals we accomplish during each decade, the fewer cancer and blood pressure screenings will be necessary during the next decade. Playing the game of life with an accomplished record creates fewer qualms when pulled from the game. At age 75, will I still concern myself with preventing heart disease as a cause of death? A colonoscopy is generally recommended at age 50. At what age do I decline the test in lieu of living out the remainder of life without a "shitload" of doctor follow-ups and diagnoses?

Moving the dialogue forward with age gives credence to patients proclaiming they are no longer being treated for a particular disease. Permission is also granted for not screening for additional illness. My certainty of being right gives credence to my motto of leaving well enough alone until I am sick enough to die. Advance Care Directives provide options for refusing feeding tubes, dialysis catheters, blood products and antibiotics if in a persistent vegetative state. Do we apply the same permission to be granted in refusing disease screening and treatment while in a conscious state? Does the strategic thinking in refusing certain treatment as part of the overall game plan occur during overtime or in the present moment?

The best time to hear how smart we are and discover lies within our hearts occurs while spontaneously conversing with others. Seemingly, those statements we make to or about others are often direct reflections of ourselves. How much of the conversation do we listen to while giving advice to our parents? By age 45, many of us are confronting our parents about end-of-life issues. How many of us take our own advice, incorporating this into our own Advance Care Directives? The feelings of helplessness experienced in attempting to assist our parents foreshadows the helplessness we will likely confront at the end of our lives. It never becomes easier with age.

Personally, a "get out of jail free" card is more important to me than a health insurance card. There is no guaranty that ensures maintaining good health; therefore, I prefer to establish a guaranty for how my life will end in the event my health declines. Frequently, dying is thought to be an out-of-body experience that tends to escape reality and certainty. Confusion keeps patients, families and physicians at odds. What should we do? What would they want? A clear directive stacks the deck with a "get out of jail free" card. The commencement of Advance Care Directives declares wishes along with instructions as to when to play this "get out of jail free" card.

WISH 9:

Pre-Wish for Peace

"We have a difficulty breathing in Room 11," the charge nurse announces. I enter the room and greet a frail elderly man gasping for breath, his wife and two children at his side. The patient has end-stage COPD that appears to be reaching a finale. I ask about his requiring previous ventilator support and the family denies his breathing ever being this bad. If I place him on a ventilator, the possibility of him ever being weaned off is doubtful. Family members' facial expressions appear to be pleading with me to save his life now and ask questions later. A pressurized oxygen mask is placed on the patient while I order the administration of bronchodilators, steroids, and a sedative. I figuratively hold my breath.

Fortunately, this patient responds well to treatment and is in no immediate need of a ventilator. With the situation having become less dire, I probe further into his wishes regarding life support. His daughter then decides to step forward as the self-appointed spokesperson. Initially, she seem to be biting her lip while biding for more time with her father. She admits that his wish is not to be placed on a ventilator. She must have known that I was literally seconds away from doing just that upon his arrival. To reinforce that the certainty of being right would be granted to her father in the future, I suggest she be more upfront about her father's wishes.

When an elderly or chronically ill patient presents to the Emergency Department with a decreased level of consciousness or difficulty breathing, I attempt to ascertain if the patient has any wishes. My treatment goals are geared toward giving patients the best care possible while respecting their wishes. Typically, providers are expected to treat all patients equally in the delivery of healthcare. Patients generally take for granted that they will receive best standard practice. However, if the steamroller of a particular illness happens to level a patient, I prefer to help lift the patient's spirit through granting final wishes rather than proceeding with futile protocols or procedures that only serve to prolong the inevitable.

A thought-provoking conversation occurred with another family whose mother was receiving palliative care for bone marrow cancer. Palliative care can be either aggressive or conservative depending on patients' wishes. This patient was somnolent from an overwhelming infection. The family was aware that the end was near, but did not expect it anytime soon. The plan was to address the situation properly as lab results were posted. It became increasingly clear that the patient was in need of aggressive life support and I posed this question to family members: "Are we going to allow nature to take its course or do you prefer to determine the course of action?" Did this family care to shoulder the responsibility of when their mother might be taken off life support? They elected to acquiesce to Mother Nature.

My Advance Care Directive acknowledges my inevitable death and establishes guidelines for my care. It acknowledges that there will be a combination of unforeseen circumstances and natural causes to take into account. Few people wish to accept responsibility for ending their own lives. When I inquire about end-of-life wishes, I am generally deferred to some medical record with the statement, "You have all of that on file." I particularly chuckle when elderly men insist, "My wife makes all those decisions." Certainly, patients have wishes. Like birthday wishes, these are frequently secret or filed away somewhere, left for others to guess what they might be and where they might be hidden. Beyond the hem and haw, I am certain that heartfelt desires are important, directive and require notation in a wish list.

The elderly are reluctant to age, but they acknowledge that the alternative is death. People proceed from wishing to not grow old to wishing to not die. While not eager to die, I continue to explore the alternative possibility of actually being able to welcome death. Witnessing many patients' plights during their numerous attempts to defy death has convinced me that the agony often endured in the process may not be worth staying alive. When the alternative to death becomes an extended hospital stay followed by a prolonged period in an extended-care facility, the question of which is better arises. Procrastination while dying easily leads to end-of-life wishes being circumvented rather than realized.

It is understood that when patients arrive in the Emergency Department, they come with the unspoken wish to not die. However, I do believe that in the back of most patients' minds is the list of events, circumstances and situations in which their preference would be to die. Serious predicaments often begin with health problems that we may choose to ignore, eventually progressing to chronic illness that we no longer wish to endure. I have observed diabetic patients live through a multitude of undue complications, prompting my directive to be in a diabetic coma before having more than one limb removed. However, we need wishes that take precedence in determining how and when we are excused from prolonging agony and suffering.

One convenient rationalization about wishes is that they are dependent upon the circumstances. There are many common situations at the end of life that are unthinkable—making rational wishes default to wishful thinking. When presenting treatment options to a patient, this dialogue often triggers false hopes that the physician is actually capable of reversing the progression of a chronic illness or even the process of dying. We cannot avoid death any more than we can avoid heartache while approaching the end of life. A question for the ages is, "How does it all end?" Writing about life ending from the perspective of dying in peace is preferable.

Among the many definitions of peace, one that strikes me as most impactful is peace defined as *deceased*. The all-too-common struggle of holding on and letting go simultaneously while in the throes of death does not embody peace. I observe the same conflict in my parents reflected in most elderly patients admitted to the ED. They are experiencing ongoing internal struggles between aging bodies and determined minds that wish to hold on as long as possible instead of being capable of stating, "I am at peace with dying."

I can hear my father readily saying, "I'm at peace because I have no choice." Wouldn't it be better if peace inspired his choice? Peace being the absence of malice might save him from the internal hostility and frustration that propels him to keep moving forward, resulting in falls, head injuries and ED visits. Peace serves as an invitation for more periods of respite rather than options and more freedom than duty. With limited freedom, particularly for someone like my father—confined to a wheelchair and being refrained from smoking—uncertainty clouds peace of mind. For him to embrace a wish to die amid the certainty of his situation not improving, I imagine a peace plan in the making that averts any battle cry.

Being at peace is not a steady state, but an invitation to let go of existing struggles both within ourselves and in our relationships. When not at peace within ourselves, we often attempt to please others to the extreme of losing our own peace and/or freedom. Actions are often averted that we know to be right as we simultaneously diminish our own self-worth. Self-esteem aids in asserting self-control. While we are apt to put up a fight when faced with insult or injury, a peace plan commences with the prospect of self-control. This peace initiative unfolds through finding contentment in the moment of discontent with the personal resolve for having wishes seed contentment.

Dying peacefully must be mindful. We are apt to become engaged in a war on terror while dying, as our bodies seemingly become our own worst enemies. Caution is needed about engaging in any war on terror without first developing an exit strategy. Like a deer caught in headlights, we may potentially become paralyzed and unable to cross to the other side of the road. When it comes to dying, an exit strategy pre-plans this acknowledgement and combats the notion of being our own worst enemy. The ideas in this book offer several means to control this war on terror by declaring specific wishes in order to make peace for ourselves. Preempting this war in a cause for peace allows people to rest in peace.

Advance Care Directives create the wherewithal for wishes to clearly be known and communicated. Collecting our thoughts and wishes in any type of near death experience is challenging. In the disorientation of turmoil, we may begin to wonder, "Where am I?" Illness or injury may not have been planned, but the endpoint we seek would be driven by wishes. It is extremely difficult to resolve exactly where we are while in a state of confusion.

How is individuality maintained amid family members' emotional demands when confronted with death? When Plan A is to live strong and die at home, Plan B is instituted when the prophylactic shatters and living at home is no longer an option. When the plan to live forever places all our eggs in one basket, what happens when one egg cracks? The inevitable crack in the egg destroys the promise of life, creating a rather messy situation.

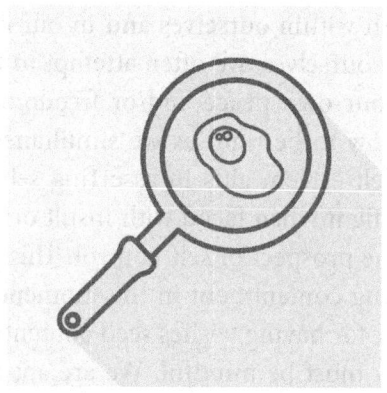

Separating the yolk from the egg white is a contemplative practice of keeping both the yolk and certainty of our wishes intact throughout the process of dying. The white protoplasm of the egg serves to protect our survival. It supports the yolk that contains dignity. Contained in the yolk are wishes for peace, harmony and freedom. The core of these wishes is easy to appreciate, but slippery to grasp when having to separate from life. Opposites attract in the crucible of this world; a shell that commingles a joint purpose. The law of physics deems that for every action there is an equal and opposite reaction. Survival potentially corrupts peace, harmony and freedom. Wishing to die or not die involves juggling the yolk back and forth. To extract the intact yolk with the certainty of being right requires separating ourselves from the engulfing white matter of self-preservation.

The preexisting wish to avert death is simple human nature. In the past, preexisting health conditions required payment of higher insurance premiums or individuals were simply denied benefits altogether. However, having preexisting wishes to die amid certain medical conditions becomes extremely useful when outlined in Advance Care Directives. Wishes are suspect in the face of serious illness. Any wish to die may be potentially discounted or completely denied on the grounds that the patient is too despondent, distraught or depressed, thereby not demonstrating the competency to refuse treatment. During almost every shift I work in the ED, I encounter patients who state, "I wish to leave now." These patients can only be released if I deem them competent.

Competency is viewed as the ability to make "proper" decisions based upon what the majority of society believes to be right. When confronted with serious illness—or injury, what becomes right is to avenge the wrong—for patients to be treated right and hopefully recover. Wishes become one-sided when compared to what everyone else does in similar situations. Very few individuals are allowed to die expeditiously. I equate dying peacefully with being able to die expeditiously. We may encounter illnesses to battle, but I believe we choose our own battles.

Wishes expressed in Advance Care Directives confront and comfort us in precarious life-threatening situations. Often in retrospect, caregivers wonder if the care their loved ones received might have been handled differently or more expeditiously. Severe illness does not afford us as much time as we would like in coming to terms with death. We cannot always choose to die on our own time. However, Advance Care Directives outline the amount of time we prefer to live and need to express how "patient" we choose to be—or not.

A well-thought-out plan is comforting when confronted with a serious injury or terminal illness. There is also comfort in defining a terminal condition in our own terms, not solely by diagnoses. If becoming quadriplegic, does the person's mind accept this way of being or is there a document that provides a meaningful escape to the confinement? When the mind deteriorates from Alzheimer's disease, is there a documented provision that allows the body to match the mind's demise? What does the heart wish for and withhold from the body when the mind cannot relay the message? When illness ends life as we know it, we have the option to treat the new illness or allow life to end in peace.

An elderly man was deeply concerned that his wife with dementia was not sleeping well at night and that she might have sleep apnea. The doctor had ordered a sleep study that would confirm the diagnosis, but would it be treated? It is difficult at best for most people to sleep while on CPAP (Continuous Positive Airway Pressure) machines. For a confused patient, the sensation of being smothered at night would probably be insufferable. Patients and their families might be encouraged to try out the "new normal" associated with advancing treatment on a trial basis—within reason and without creating additional struggles. Well-thought-out plans rightfully contain escape clauses from treatment that may not ensure peace of mind.

To be forthright in Advance Care Directives is to be purposefully introspective. Introspection acknowledges becoming heart-centered, allowing an exchange of potentially narrow-minded wishes for those that are more preordained and heartfelt. An Advance Care Directive that is inclusive of wishes commences a journey along the path of being heart-centered. Exploring wishes in the context of terminal illness consciously or unconsciously brings us to a fork in the road. Standing at this juncture, Advance Care Directives may promote leading patients down the road less traveled by implying that less is more. Less intervention supports the greater acceptance of death.

The charade of deception can become quite rampant at the end of life. There are patients who prefer everyone, including their doctors, pretend they are not dying. Others want a definitive statement of how much longer they will be alive. Most people prefer to speak truth to power regarding their human rights. Truth gives power to people who stand firm against anyone or anything that might have power over them, whether an authority figure, doctor or disease. Will our end-of-life wishes bring power to our lives? Life comprised of pretenses becomes a travesty, distortion or sham while patients become mere shadows of themselves. How we speak truth to power emerges from the soul or what I perceive to be the dream weaver of wishes.

WISH 10:

Pre-Stamp Three Coins in the Fountain

Debunking the myth that doctors are capable of saving all lives, I would rather sell people on the idea of having a genie in a bottle who grants three wishes before anything like an incurable disease occurs. Before preparing Advance Care Directives, people need to dwell on their wishes that the heart desires now and at the end of life. As much as Advance Care Directives are intended to express personal wishes, I cannot remember the last time I wished for a feeding tube, dialysis or a ventilator.

Many times advance care treatments listed on directives shame patients into doing the right things for the wrong reasons. The certainty of being right occurs when wishes come true. The certainty of being right selects the top three wishes that grant truth to power.

In general, stamping our top wishes onto three coins to be tossed into the fountain supports universal truths and personal well-being. Naturally, wishes need to address the moment, aligning with personal truth in order to achieve peace. In being given the mission of expressing three wishes, these wishes become convictions providing both certainty and direction.

What is first and foremost in my mind and in the hearts of most Americans are the immortal words of Patrick Henry: *Give me liberty or give me death.* Freedom is not only paramount to the U.S. Constitution, but also to my personal sense of well-being. In its construct, my Advance Care Directive incorporates more freedom than entrapment. Generally, freedom is appreciated by having more choices; however, more options can sometimes create confusion. If surgery is the best treatment, but surgery is not an option, freedom of choice is curtailed. When choices are limited and I no longer am capable of living semi-independently, I wish for freedom from having my life prolonged.

Certainty stems from a pledge of loyalty, conviction and allegiance. Like the Pledge of Allegiance, the commencement of my Advance Care Directive promotes devotion to myself, seeking an end to life with *liberty and justice for all*. With adrenaline-pumping uncertainty, it figuratively places my hand over my heart in deference to freedom and symbolizes the promise to ease worry. When death is imminent, I stand by an advance care pledge asserting eminent domain in lieu of any Patient's Bill of Rights. Justice lies in my freedom, not in conformity to standards.

My second wish is—*Respect my dignity by allowing me free choice.* I wish that healthcare providers include no medical intervention as being acceptable while still being afforded comfort care. When dying, I prefer other people give me the benefit of the doubt regarding my certainty of being right about wishing to pass. When patients present to the Emergency Department stating, "I think I'm dying"—their claim should be listened to and respected as them being conscious about it and having a choice in the matter. Similarly, I intend to listen and discern the difference between those caregivers who support my passing or oppose it—inasmuch—identifying those who honor my dignity.

My third wish begs *Show Me the Mercy*. I realize physicians are often expected to discuss options with patients, but I remember my mother saying: "If you don't have anything nice to say, don't say anything at all." I need physicians to spare me the life-support verbiage and *show me the mercy*. The certainty of death sets the stage for suffering to end. If fatally wounded on the battlefield, my dying wish would be, "Just shoot me!" My Advance Care Directive stores generous rounds of sedative ammunition. I wish Clint Eastwood to be at my bedside, demonstrating the same mercy he did in *Million Dollar Baby*, along with the encouragement of *Dirty Harry*, "Go ahead, make my day."

When wishing to shower mercy onto the dying, physicians frequently butt up against Advance Care Directives that, in effect, issue restraining orders against doing just that. The presumption that people wish everything be done to prolong life leaves little room for providing mercy. I wish mercy to remain foremost, particularly as my end nears. The less time I have on earth, the less emphasis I prefer to place on any means to sustain life. I respect the essential goodness of healthcare providers who may want to attempt to prolong my life. However, my Advance Care Directive will serve to lessen their accountability in regard to what is deemed medically necessary with the insistence they be blessed for showing mercy. *Blessed are the merciful, for they will be shown mercy* (Mathew 5:7).

WISH 11:

Pre-Ordain Healthcare Proxy

On the heels of a colleague's death at the age of 49, I overheard the registration clerk in the ED ask a 46-year-old man if he wished to designate a medical power of attorney. He laughed the question off with the glib statement, "No, I don't need one of those." I could not help but wonder what he was thinking in not wishing to have Clint Eastwood nearby and ready to pull the plug if needed. I wondered if he had life insurance or if he was simply cavalier with anything regarding his mortality. It seems reasonable that a responsible person at that age would have a life insurance policy, particularly if his life contributes to the support of others. Just as the responsible act of having a designated driver when incapacitated or impaired—grants our loved ones peace of mind, the same holds true regarding our end-of-life wishes.

Death can occur at any given moment. Therefore, a designated driver is always necessary to safeguard dignity. Few people actually ever assign a medical power of attorney (POA) or healthcare proxy. This person will speak on behalf of our end-of-life wishes if we are unable to do so. However, those emotionally tied and indebted to us may have difficulty upholding wishes that support death. Choosing a cohort who is willing, ready and able to honor and facilitate our wishes is frequently preferable to a spouse who has promised to always love, honor and cherish.

Family ties often prevent patients from dying with dignity—as they may overtly express their loved ones' wishes from a personal perspective and righteous indignation. For a physician to suggest that a patient be allowed to die is blasphemous to the profession and is easier to broach with a reasonable mediator than with overly emotional family members. Most medical POA's stand in defense of prolonging life rather than defining what it means for the person to die with dignity. When my sister requested I be her medical POA, I respectfully declined due to the miles between us. She retorted by raising my awareness that the distance factor was what she was seeking: "I just need someone to pull the plug and I know you will do it."

Creating and maintaining healthy emotional boundaries between patients, caregivers and healthcare providers is the responsibility of the medical POA. One of the primary goals for the medical POA is to maintain reasonability and certainty when the situation derails emotionally. In addition, the certainty of the healthcare proxy being right is stronger when medical options—that only serve to prolong lives when patients have pre-determined their will to die—are cleared from the table.

The certainty of being right is similar to pre-planning a final itinerary aboard a cruise ship. While anticipating this end-of-life journey, it is wise to have a pre-packed disaster preparedness kit. Patients frequently regret not bringing an overnight bag when unexpectedly admitted to the hospital. Keeping an attaché of advance care getaway papers, comprise the boarding pass for the virtual cruise ship. The joy of cruising is derived from being relieved of many of life's obligations. Advance Care Directives make the early boarding process much easier. Envisioning smooth sailing as a final wish is one way to encourage hearing *bon voyage* from loved ones sooner than later.

Bon voyage is a salutation rarely appreciated at the end of life. Tragically, a man I was caring for had severed ties with his daughter who lived in another part of the country twenty years prior. On his deathbed he remorsefully cried to her over the phone. Sensitive to his situation and fear, she struggled to arrange for a flight that would allow her to be by his side. His contrition and certainty of making the situation right with his daughter was admirable. Leaving unfinished business until the end challenged both of us to question our responsibilities in matters presumably close to his heart.

It is important to say "Good-bye." It's hard to comprehend why people appear too busy or fearful to say it. Hawaiians encompass the entire end of life dialogue in one word: "Aloha!" Translated as meaning hello, good-bye, love, affection, peace, honor, compassion and mercy—this can be offered to anyone at any time—it does not need to be reserved solely for the end of life. Most people are stuck in the belief that there are no appropriate words to comfort the dying, or that they lack the capacity to express the depth of their love. Every person's life is a gift, and as with any gift, the certainty of being right comes across through attaching thoughtful words or sentiments with a card. When becoming sentimental, a shift occurs from being self-absorbed to heart-centered. Survivors feel compelled to say something to their dying loved ones. However, it becomes less trying when the heart awakens and relates its message.

Ideally, when Advance Care Directives become activated, advance notice is given to family members to express their feelings to the patient while providing sustenance for the end-of-life journey. When conversations remain unspoken or incomplete, the impetus is to reverse the process of dying and prolong life. What normally is left unsaid is a "thank you," a debt, an apology or simply continuity. When continuity of the relationship is the motivation, people need to *pause, center and shift* from perpetuating the relationship to honoring the perpetuity of love. Unfortunately, sometimes we live with the regret of the last conversation being an argument, or that we were too choked up to speak; however, it is never too late to realize thanks through remembrance. I practiced what I preached through a heartfelt letter to my mother on her 88th birthday (Appendix I).

Saying "good-bye" at the end of life is bittersweet, yet necessary. Otherwise, plans become waylaid and the cruise ship may depart without a farewell. It is easy to become hung up and strung out over others needing to express departing words. Consequently, a person is requested to be kept alive on life support until family and friends have all had an opportunity for closure. My directive includes the wish for others to find their own means of letting me go without keeping me alive artificially. Separated by many miles and not in a life-or-death situation, I created a way to say goodbye to my father on his 83rd birthday. The time seemed right to take the opportunity to celebrate his life and extend the wish of "many happy returns" for his future with a note of thanks (Appendix II).

Having bid farewell, what emerged was both the indifference of needing to be present at his death and yet maintaining an emotional attachment to his life. I continue to be an ardent defender of his "passing"—passing on doctor visits and passing on the need to be resuscitated. As his tour of civilian duty approaches the end, my intention is for him to be honorably discharged. Subsequent visits have provided goodies for his journey. The deathbed needs to be reserved as a place for comfort—with personal good-byes already expressed and put to rest. The talking point that I remind myself of has become, "Dad, you've done enough and I'm grateful for what you have done. I do not expect you to do anything more."

Some people are possessed to literally drag a dying person into the Emergency Department and insist that more be done. In most of these situations there has been a breakdown in communication between the patient and family members. Partially, it is the patient's fault because they have not previously had the wherewithal to declare, "I'm done." However, family members who disallow patients from openly expressing their fears and wishes while approaching death are also at fault. Inevitably, patients and family members alike attempt to shift much of the decision-making responsibility about being finished in life onto physicians' shoulders.

Are we prepared to be free to enjoy the rest of our days in peace? Frequently, family members are consumed with wishing to do the right thing before life ends. Why not make the end of our life right by splurging on something perceived as well deserved. The Make-A-Wish Foundation grants this experience by fulfilling a dream of a child with a terminal illness. As dying patients are apt to regress to becoming childlike, perhaps a family's focus is better directed toward fulfilling a wish rather than solely supporting a wish to die. Dignity is centered in the certainty of a wish, allowing the heart to be lifted when the wish comes true. Wishes are not magic; magic is happenstance. Having a wish fulfilled is uplifting and received with critical acclaim.

WISH 12:

Pre-Meditate Critical Thinking

Crucial, life-threatening situations are addressed by calling 911 and receiving critical care. Terminal, end-of-life illness is addressed by critical thinking with consideration given to comfort care. Terminal situations are subject to emotional overlay and confusion. Clear, rational thinking requires collecting and prioritizing intentions during a decisive moment. During a terminal event, patients take a turn for the worse and are thrust into a downward spiral. Adding insult to injury, they are often bombarded by the shame inherent in dying. Loss of confidence and disgrace are only truly regained through the process of critical thinking.

Against the headwinds of end-stage COPD, Roger was perspiring and purse-lip breathing. Within the last month, he had undergone surgery for colon cancer and had a doctor appointment that day to discuss treatment options for his ongoing prostate cancer. He understood the radiation implant had burned his prostate, but the cancer remained active based on an elevated lab test. Having maxed out his treatment options for end-stage COPD, it was curious that he was expending energy on being cancer free when his lung disease would likely cause his death. A sedative to relieve the tension in his chest. After a short while, Roger claimed he had not felt this well in months. Why did he continued to fight each battle on all fronts? I hoped to unravel the noose that was choking off his ability to breathe comfortably.

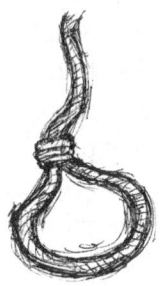

Probing further, I discovered he and his wife had moved to Arizona from California in an effort to save their daughter's marriage. While meddling in others' lives, he seemed to have little control over his own. In the past, he balanced stress by playing in a band. He still had his wind instruments, but was spending more time recovering from medical procedures than rehearsing for performances. By jamming more illness on his plate than jamming with his band, he could no longer breathe comfortably. In the wake of his Titanic repeatedly crashing into the iceberg with each illness, he was intent on boarding the next lifeboat while his heart's desire might be to play with the orchestra. There are many parts to the composition of life; critical thinking advocates playing the part we prefer.

Roger had good intentions, but his thought processes did not appear to be aiding his certainty. Good intentions naturally oblige us to do more, presumably by some unwritten rule of law. Critical thinking challenges this rule of law with an abiding rule of thumb. The rule of thumb provides a rough estimation that is not based on science, nor is it reliable in every situation or person. It is a practical rule that recalls values and makes determinations more personal. Applying our rule of thumb to commencing Advance Care Directives makes them more personal and less cookbook.

As I connect the certainty of being right to recalling values, my Advance Care Directive commences with this line of thinking. With any illness or injury we are apt to lose the value of being human—along with perceived value judgments regarding the reality of what is to be considered and addressed. In deciding if any claim is true, we need to apply critical thinking. The defining directive and personal objective inherent to critical thinking is to *clarify goals, examine assumptions, discern hidden values, evaluate evidence, accomplish actions and assess conclusions.*[2] When patients give "informed consent," it is presumed that they have considered all their options. Unfortunately, it quickly ricochets back to the doctor's expertise. Critical thinking provides preconceived answers to impossible questions asked of patients.

For any report or Advance Care Directive to be considered complete, it must emphasize rationality. A checklist of the Five W's must be answered:

__Who
__What
__Where
__When
__Why

Five W's provide the complete story and aid critical thinking in conjunction with honoring wishes. Routinely, these five questions regarding acute illness are expected to be answered by the doctor. With the Five W's being supplanted on top of our three wishes and having the tables turned, I cannot imagine being granted three wishes and then allowing the doctor to determine who, what, where, when and why.

In essence, having three wishes clarifies goals, creating the game plan for an end-of-life strategy. Patients' wishes can be explored by asking, "What is the goal?" Is it living to be 100 years old, or to know when the time has come to die? Critical thinking invokes the Five W's, which helps patients define goals and assist in the commencement of Advance Care Directives:

- Who is in charge *examines assumptions.*
- What *hidden values* are brought to light?
- "Where's is the beef" in *evaluating the evidence*?
- When is it necessary to *accomplish actions*?
- Why *assess conclusions* if no consideration is given to the right to die?

Most living wills are created from the mindset of wishing to live rather than die. A woman who preferred not to receive dialysis had a family that insisted she have dialysis, The contest of wills between preserving her self-determination and the family's desire to prolong her life was detrimental to all. This patient was more than capable of making her own decisions but the family discounted her ability to reason because of a recent stroke. The collective *you*, as in family, generally speaks loudly when life is at stake. However, the contemplative *you* may have a very different desire and voice needing to be heard and honored. Who was truly speaking for this patient's wishes became quite confusing. Advance Care Directives can allay this type of confusion.

Most people wish to live, becoming perplexed by this perceived intruder that takes over our minds with the inconceivable will to die. As the end draws near, we deliberate and weigh life support options against having the will to live or die. There is no critical thinking given to Advance Care Directives that reiterate expressions of "living wills." Each of us begins life with the will to live. However, Advance Care Directives are most valuable when offering guidance in assessing the who, what, when, where and why of withdrawing or withholding care—commencing a will to die.

Who is in charge of examining assumptions?

As we *examine assumptions* within Advance Care Directives, I am reminded of one of The Four Agreements based upon the writings of Don Miguel Ruiz: *Don't Make Any Assumptions.*[3] The question of **Who** violates this agreement is the patient who assumes doctors will fix everything and miracles actually happen. Reinforcing this assumption, I happened upon the headline, "Newborn Baby Declared Dead Wakes Up." If declared brain dead, life support can be withdrawn quickly. However, while in a persistent vegetative state, lower brain stem reflexes are retained that can trigger cycles of being seemingly awake or asleep. These patients have no awareness of anything around them, yet assumptions will be plentiful. Arguably, caregivers wish to sustain life in this situation based upon the assumption that the person is actually still there.

From the perspective of being in a persistent vegetative state, Advance Care Directives pose a number of menu selections including liquid concoctions, access to the oxygen bar, finger foods or stomach tubes, entrees infused with blood products and served with an optional side of organic antibiotics.

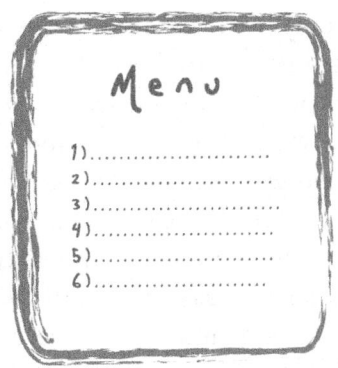

Faith can be strong enough to order room service as a full "Course in Miracles" that one day may heed the command from Jesus to *Rise, take up your mat and walk* (John 5:8). A testament to faith is based on beliefs formulated from assumptions passed on from generations through millenniums. Advance Care Directives seem to follow the same perception. Make no assumptions; there is a grand desire to be walking proof that God exists.

Many people seem to prefer Advance Care Directives that leave the door open to interventions that instill miracles cures. As God works in mysterious ways, this type of uncertainty can drive patients and everyone else involved in their care crazy. While Advance Care Directives may aspire to be inclusive of God's plan, they may also include the wish to remove a feeding tube when miracles are not forthcoming. In the context of unwavering faith while hoping for the best, are people still responsible for planning for the worst-case scenario? Is faith allowed to wane while people advance in age or after spending weeks, months or years in a persistent vegetative state?

A healthy skepticism regarding healthcare professionals needs to be maintained by patients and family members in all encounters. The "already always listening" assumed by many physicians is that patients wish to be treated the same and will respond to standard practice. In divergent situations, some patients prefer alternative measures, no treatment, or prefer to simply obtain a work excuse. Some patients insist upon a thorough workup; others are content to swallow a pill. There are those patients whose only need is to receive reassurance that their time and mine is not being wasted. How patients wish to be treated remains a diagnostic mystery. Clearly, patients need to be more conscious, upfront and honest about expectations and assumptions.

Don't make assumptions increases awareness regarding potential maltreatment that occurs in the zeal and mindset of doing no harm through ordering well-intentioned tests. In reality, many tests result in false positives. There is also an assumption that most patients view the "good doctor" as a good humanitarian. However, there are good doctors who capitalize on patients' illness, with the doctor's capital accruing through coercion and the financial charges of treating any and all illness. There may be a conflict of interest within the good doctor as the good businessperson. The conundrum in this situation is that patients often feel better or more worthy when they assume the money being spent is all for their benefit.

Typically, patients freely assume they know very little about medicine and the *all-knowing* doctor knows everything. Frequently, as knowledge about a patient or illness increases, more mystery becomes apparent. The adage about knowing more and understanding less proves to be humbling for most physicians. What is initially taught as the correct treatment may eventually be cited as the wrong course of action. The certainty of a particular treatment may actually be more an afterthought than forethought. Nevertheless, this does not excuse having certainty and dignity remain foremost to making decisions. While assuming many patients know very little, there are times when they catch me off guard with insightful statements that redirect my thinking.

The challenge in making assumptions begins with knowing every person will eventually die; yet there are many who assume that illness is not supposed to kill them. *Don't Make Assumptions* reminds me of having to guess the answers on a final exam when homework was not complete or an assignment is returned marked in red ink. We spend much time suffering when unprepared to fill in the blanks. When dying with dignity is an assumption, the consequence of additional suffering is often imposed. It is difficult to distinguish assumptions from certainty without prior examination. The path to dignity is not an assumption, but one that is established by certainty.

What hidden values are brought to light?

The question of **What** to do in matters of life and death as outlined in Advance Care Directives occurs through *discerning hidden values.* The values I hold close to my heart are easily shrouded by the predominance of inalienable rights. Among these are life, liberty and the pursuit of happiness. Many of us share the same values perceived as rights, but prioritize them differently in order to attain a place in heaven. I grew up admiring the Gale Sayers' motto, "The Lord is first, my friends are second, and I am third."[4] Without giving it much thought at the time, this order seemed reasonable, particularly; as I was heavily invested in giving the Lord his due. Moreover, my lack of self-esteem never allowed me to be cast in the leading role.

The specifics of Advance Care Directives are largely dictated by a personal inventory of life values. With God being first, my Advance Care Directive would theoretically be determined by the Lord or the "law," conforming to lawful and acceptable practices. Before approaching the age of 40, I was reevaluating priorities in my life. A close friend shared the life values inventory he had received from his therapist, with instructions to identify my top five. Surprisingly, God did not top my list. Instead, I identified personal freedom as what I valued most in life. The idea of being stripped of my personal freedom by means of imprisonment would virtually kill me no matter how much I trusted God or cared for my family.

As reflected in living my life, the remaining top values in descending order were financial stability, health and fitness, family relationships, and spiritual well-being. In some respects this placed God in more of a supportive role, allowing me increased latitude for personal free will to become the deciding factor. Just as I understood God to be first on my list as a child, I realized my values changed as I evolved as a person. I recall that many relationships built upon certain convictions amounted to feelings that did not hold steadfast. Presently, my Advance Care Directive is designed to ensure my personal freedom as primary—not have it deferred to the "Big Guy" or some "better half."

A personal inventory of hidden values is a vital wellspring of resources to be drawn upon while creating Advance Care Directives. Personal life values serve as ideals that we strive to attain. Resources may actually appear limited until they are identified and recruited as being useful for our lives. Illness tends to catch us off guard and subvert our values, resulting in decisions being made through insinuation and subjugation. People often regress to childlike uncertainty with limited coping resources and rely heavily on the support of other adults. After maturing to adulthood, the goal is to quiet the inner child by drawing upon personal values as our greatest resources. The following list represents life values worth considering when creating Advance Care Directives:

Achievement	Belonging
Concern for the Environment	Concern for Others
Creativity	Financial Prosperity
Health and Activity	Humility
Independence	Loyalty to Family or Group
Privacy	Responsibility
Scientific Understanding	Spirituality

I am able to repeatedly look at this list and ascertain those values that are operative in patients' lives. When I approach reevaluating my existing Advance Care Directive, this is the list I contemplate at each mid-decade birthday. Becoming wiser with age, I realize the overall aspiration to value life in general requires decided specificity. If confined to an extended-care facility without personal freedom, I am less inclined to believe that my life would hold any value.

Once specific values are identified, they serve as the foundation from which decisions are based. In the face of terminal illness the task is to remain focused on life values in lieu of special interest parties. As Vice President Joe Biden states, "Don't tell me what you value, show me your budget and I'll tell you what you value." I believe values from any inventory list will our become self-evident on Judgment Day. Standing before God, will life choices be consistent with values that reflect being true to ourselves?

"This above all: to thine own self be true" are Shakespeare's words that hold value. The certainty of being right will continue to torment us amidst divergent ideologies existing in the world. The certainty of being right occurs through self-realization of what we value. The hidden value of "to thine own self be true" is the desire to die peacefully, not necessarily by assisted suicide or active euthanasia. Typically, the topic of euthanasia is discussed in hushed, quiet conversations that take place when patients are dying. Examining thoughts and beliefs about euthanasia explores its potential value and the personal values we express in life, whether it condemns or dispenses mercy.

The quote that gives credence to being true to ourselves is provided by the ancient Greek philosopher, Epictetus: "It's not what happens to you, but how you react to it that matters." The reaction reveals values. "To be or not to be, that is the question" Shakespeare poses. Is it better to live or not live? The answer to this question resides in whether we are true to ourselves. Countless patients present to the Emergency Department with both subtle and not-so-subtle claims of "I'm dying here." Some die before their time and others live on borrowed time. How many of these people remain true to their values?

"Where's is the beef" in evaluating the evidence?

Where the point of no return is crossed becomes answered through *evaluating the evidence* and examining our conscience. When the evidence does not support quality of life, do we have an exit strategy? I was dumbfounded by a patient with metastatic colon cancer who believed he was cured when two metastatic lesions in his lungs were removed by a surgeon. I wondered what evidence supported his claim of being cancer free. Once cancer spreads, it springs up like weeds in the landscape of the body while potentially lying beneath the radar. He was admitted to the ED later with horrific back pain after a chiropractor completed an adjustment and was immediately awakened to the horror of his spine being riddled with cancer.

As evidenced by that conversation, I realized that I only get bits and pieces of patients' stories. I do not believe the physician misled his patient, but like other patients, he seized and held onto any crumb of hope. Where do we place hope in the scheme of awareness and where is trust regarding the prospect of certainty? Do we aspire to have hope but err on the side of evidence or uncertainty? What becomes apparent is how ready most people are to embrace hope while discounting scientific evidence. This patient maintained a wonderful smile despite the misery of metastatic disease. The hope of reclaiming his cancer-free status provided him positive energy, but there was little clear, rational thinking in play.

Critical thinking requires an evaluation of the evidence independent of the doctor. From the doctor's perspective, any evaluation of the evidence might undermine his/her credibility. When everything goes well in surgery, patients have the best surgeon in the world; however, if surgery goes awry, the doctor is awful. Doctors hope for the best outcome, rarely mentioning complications that would suggest the patient has the wrong physician. Trust, but verify information provided by the doctor is particular necessary in dealing with terminal illness. Let the evidence speak for itself and remain unclouded by wishful thinking. There is a reason why terminal illness is terminal and why it is imperative for evidence to add certainty to the decision-making process.

With each presidential election cycle, Ronald Reagan's question pops up: "Are you better off today than you were four years ago?" The question at the end of life becomes: Are you better off today than you were four months or four days ago? Countless families discount the evidence of today as a patient progressively deteriorates. Inevitably, I hear, "You would not believe who this patient was several months ago." Let the record show that this patient was previously healthy while allowing the evidence to show what has now become of the patient. Certainty becomes more evident and reliable when patients and family members choose to stay in the moment.

When is it necessary to accomplish actions?

More than simply words, Advance Care Directives *accomplish action*. The steps we take merge consciously with the interrogative of **When** they are taken. When does "enough already" become complete with a directive that lists the action to be taken when patients declare being done? When do we support mission accomplished in lieu of mission impossible in attempting to defy death? Normally, a peace treaty would be signed and fighting would cease once a mission is completed. Through Advance Care Directives, we seek to accomplish action for or against withholding or withdrawing treatment. Critical thinking links the notion of a peace treaty with Advance Care Directives, ascertaining and accomplishing a graceful exit at the end of life.

Uncertainty confounds end-of-life conversations and situations—patients are uncertain about what to do and doctors are uncertain about which actions to take. In this moment of confusion, dignity often lapses. Subsequent actions taken will impact dignity positively or negatively. The paradigm of Advance Care Directives needs to advocate for certainty being conferred in death, resisting the insistence that all action be taken in support of sustaining life no matter the situation. For myself, when quality of life ends I want action that accomplishes and supports my will to die. Upon crossing the finish line, any action that proposes or imposes prolonging life would sacrifice my dignity.

In accomplishing actions, what actions result from misunderstandings and words unspoken? What seems less than important in life often becomes paramount at the end of life. I am often challenged by which action is to be taken while family members and friends gather at bedside. The dignity of the patient can become usurped by any intervention I inflict upon the unenthusiastic patient, requiring the need to prolong life until family members come to grips with the situation. In comparison to the popular slogan, "Never let them see you sweat," my Advance Care Directive becomes, "never let them see me sweat on life support while gawking at my demise." When my time is up I can be held at bay until my organs are taken. Then the rest of my body may be cremated. The certainty of being right permits me to die when my time comes—not determined by others' timeframes or emotional hang-ups.

Why assess conclusions if no consideration is given to the right to die?

Critical thinking is necessary to assess conclusions, allowing for dignity to be redeemed. **Why** we repeatedly *assess conclusions* ascertains whether we are still on the right path or not. As with any lesson in life, *teach me the path to love/dignity to take* concludes with a final assessment. My certainty of being right is to be assessed by how much I am suffering and whether mercy is being granted during the process of dying. Much of my career has been spent assessing whether the forgone conclusion of one's dying actually honors the sanctity of that individual's life. Many family members insist that doctor prevent loved ones near the end of life be resuscitated. Nevertheless, I have y attempted to anticipate ways to ensure nothing be done to prolong my life when the time comes. For me, dignity is realized in passing sooner than later.

In assessing conclusions one thing to die from needs to be identified, and not a multitude of diagnoses to discover and treat. The whys and wherefores of troublesome circumstances could be overridden by simply allowing any wrongs to be viewed as acceptable life lessons, providing an opportunity to set an example. A friend told me his 92-year-old aunt was taken from the nursing home to the Emergency Department and he expressed hope that she would be admitted to the hospital for evaluation and assessment. Why was he concerning himself with her being ill when he was convinced that it was time for her to pass? The mystery of illness adds to the mystery of death; being aggressive in an assessment only added to her suffering. Assessing conclusions provides a quicker course correction and a reprieve from assessing further illnesses requiring intervention.

If ever bedridden from a stroke, I would insist that metrics—like monitoring my blood pressure, heart rhythm and lab studies—are not necessary to track or treat. I am less concerned with bedsores being treated, preferring they present evidence of my persistent vegetative state. I would be content to simply have my pain treated without looking too intently for what may be causing the pain. By streamlining my care and discontinuing any efforts to prolong life, I will expedite dying. I prefer to assess conclusions without beating around the bush. Knowing the tricks of the trade in the delivery of healthcare, a patient lessens the chance of having their dignity undermined by ambiguity.

Generally, we wish for a speedy recovery and a return to good health. However, when recovery has a poor prognosis, we can utilize this information in assessing conclusions. People usually equate a poor prognosis with the need to increase efforts to work or pray for a more positive outcome. It may be more effective to use critical thinking and having conclusions supported by a doctor. It is a rare doctor who speaks bluntly about dying. The best clue might come about by being given a poor prognosis. Most people liken a poor prognosis to being given their walking papers. Better to think of these papers as being unnecessary and have patients maintain their own personal walking papers in conjunction with a clear, concise Advance Care Directive.

A frequent lingering question posed over the course of any serious illness is "Why me?" Don Miguel Ruiz' Second Agreement is *Do Not Take Anything Personally*—even dying. This agreement negates the existential question of "Why me?" Understanding the reality that everyone must die, there is no reason to take dying personally. Of course, this is much easier said than done. In regard to death as the means to enter the kingdom of heaven, Jesus claims, *Again I say to you, it is easier for a camel to pass through the eye of a needle than for* (Mathew 19:24) . . . a person to not take death personally. To think beyond the emotional upheaval and aversion to being stuffed in a box or urn, we need to reframe the conversation along a spiritual directive that would ask, "Why not me?"

The attitude of "fake it till you make it," is an acknowledgement of having to somehow fake it till we make dying rational. Typically, how we fake it is by making stuff up. I make sense of dying by making stuff up about what may happen as I transition to the other side. In some dubious testimony regarding death and dying, we might acknowledge *the spirit is indeed willing, but the flesh is weak* (Mathew 26:41). Our spirits are willing to die, but our minds typically entertain second thoughts. The spirit, being interdependent upon the body, will still remain impersonal. The soul can embody life or leave it. The spirit, inherent to the soul, sets the course for peace. I envision this leading to some dream state allowing me to levitate beyond this life. I assess conclusions by how well my fears are calmed while in this dream state.

As we approach most gateways in life, there are admission requirements. We need to be just so tall to be allowed on this ride, really adept to get into a particular college and really sick to get admitted to the hospital. How is the end of life approached? How we walk the walk reveals how we may die. How we feel about dying is very subjective. It is imperative to take a step back and consider how we might live our lives right up to the end by creating a preamble to our Advance Care Directives.

Taking a walk down memory lane I recall attending a fundraiser and bidding on an opportunity to do a "walk on" performance in the Broadway musical *Sunset Blvd*. I carried the fascination with me of what it must be like to be on stage and in the spotlight. With no formal training, this "walk on" was my chance to be discovered, giving me a chance to be on stage, but not really be seen. Metaphorically, while taking a walk on the dark side of Sunset Boulevard during the twilight years, suddenly the floodlights at the end of the tunnel will cast an individual in the real-life adaptation of *On Death and Dying*. As written in the advance care script, the show must go on with the command performance inspired by a preamble.

PART III

...

Preamble To
Advance Care Directives

Wish 13:

Co-Mingle Denial with Consideration

Many conversations regarding health status take place outside the healthcare system. While dining with friends, a round-robin discussion occurred involving a laundry list of health issues. One friend, Randy, was serving as medical POA for his 92-year-old aunt hospitalized with intractable pain due to shingles. Randy just completed his annual physical, skin cancer screening, and was given a clean bill of health. Being proactive, he inquired about receiving the shingles vaccine.

Recently, Mike's 83-year-old father was evaluated for chest pain and a spot was discovered on his lung. Mike has hypertension, an expanding waistline and is now confronting pre-diabetes.

These ordinary medical situations are stepping stones to larger considerations regarding Advance Care Directives. This dinner conversation exemplifies how intelligent, well-educated people approach the certainty of disease along with uncertain futures. At what point do we ignore a spot on the lung? Is pre-diabetes best treated with weight loss or medication? Do we approach these situations with denial or consideration? We mutually agreed on the common refrain, "Let's wait and see; we'll cross that bridge when we come to it."

Meanwhile, the elderly aunt has reached the suspension bridge of a sagging hospital mattress. Her attending physician is questioning whether she would sign a Do Not Resuscitate (DNR) order. Randy did wish his aunt's life shortened and was unsure how to advise her. The same question had been proposed 10 years earlier. If she had signed the DNR then, her life may have been shortened, but it would have spared her insufferable pain of shingles. Her present situation was not terminal, but her life expectancy was. Randy argued that if her pain was adequately treated, why encourage her to sign a DNR? I would promptly sign a DNR if I were being transferred to a skilled-care facility. I do not foresee quality of life existing in such a location. The preamble of Advance Care Directives perceives many of us becoming stuck in denial and indecision, while dignity suggests exiting sooner and with certainty.

My friend's 83-year-old father is not unlike my father; however, I do not have any stories about recently finding condoms under my father's bed. My father is confined to a wheelchair. He had a spot on his lung investigated 15 years ago, but I would not advise that action today. He prides himself on being healthy and prefers to maintain his health through ignorance. Ignorance is bliss while others talk amongst themselves. Disease naturally occurs at this age. Do we give in to it? Despite having chest pain, Mike's father has some remaining stamina as evidenced in his condom use. I would encourage him to address the lung nodule; cardiac intervention might enhance the activities he enjoys.

Stagnation is self-defeating. Preambles envision keeping an eye out for these types of potholes while trekking down the rocky road near the end of life. Randy has a degree in psychology, teaches and practices yoga and is intent on harnessing the most from life. He is sensitive to caring for his aunt like he wishes to be treated and by taking advantage of every opportunity to remain healthy. However, he feels defeated in making end-of-life decisions for himself, much less what considerations are important for his aunt and her well-being and dignity.

When life matters, there is an obligation to sustain life to the point of actually denying aging. There are for middle-aged people who prefer not to become old, and elderly persons who deny imminent death. Could we change this conundrum and begin to honor the aging process? Growing old is never easy as many patients attest—"It's hell getting old." While taking measures and medication to prevent aging, the preamble for Advance Care Directives effectively guides the passage to becoming old, diseased and disgruntled. With foresight, positive steps and reasonable options can be taken preventively. In contrast, a wait-and-see attitude allows pre-diabetes to become diabetes, perhaps resulting in excruciating neuropathy or receiving dialysis routinely. My certainty of being right commits me to be as healthy as possible today to avoid remedial treatment in the future.

We are generally set in our ways by middle age, shaped by life experiences. Once "over the hill," are we still open to change? I observed the contrast in my two friends at dinner: Randy is completing an advanced yoga certification to help people with disabilities. Mike foolishly lets unwise eating habits get the best of his weight and his health. Both appear willing to wait and see what their futures hold. Both claim to be proactive in addressing their health. But Randy is getting in front of the proverbial eight ball while Mike is slipping behind it.

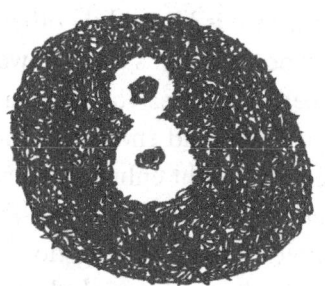

If we decide to "wait and see," at what point do we confront the future? When do we stop taking health for granted and begin taking control of our health—before or after a sudden heart attack? Why are people rarely willing to imagine the prospect and prevalence of disease when warnings about smoking, fast food consumption and the need for exercise appear everywhere? Consideration begins with an examination of conscience. Are we set for the long run and recognize what conveniences will shorten our run? Health becomes less certain after a heart attack along with questions regarding intense activities. Weight gain potentiates arthritis, affording another excuse not to exercise.

What happens in life is we experience pain, notice an abnormal lump or develop a vague sensation of not feeling right. Generally, a visit to the doctor distinguishes a quick fix from a potential setback, a chronic condition from end-stage disease. The diagnosis of terminal illness triggers enactment of Advance Care Directives. One of the first questions posed by patients upon being given bad news is, "How much time do I have?" An appropriate response might be, "How much time did you allot in your preamble and document in your Advance Care Directive?" What would be a reasonable amount of time to devote to a terminal illness? As with life-threatening situations, *timing is everything* and *time is of the essence* regarding life and death.

Whether life begins at age 40 or 50 becomes irrelevant if you divide that life into two halves: the sunny side and the lunar side. Consideration of Advance Care Directives begins with the lunar side of life, realizing personal insights at this stage of a preamble. How agile are we in the middle of life? Does agility have anything to do with dignity? By the age of 50 we are as limber as we are going to be, unless we exercise regularly. We have the choice to be flexible during our middle years, but will that choice still prevail at the end of life?

The first coping stage identified in Elisabeth Kübler-Ross' *On Death and Dying* is denial. The preamble to my Advance Care Directive considers denial to be procrastination. Despite enjoying excellent health in my midlife, my preamble considerations address the propensity to one day be like my parents. In questioning my parents' choices, I am cognizant of the potential inconsistency and uncertainty that plague life. Steps taken early in life may avert how closely we follow our parents' footsteps. Missteps and misuse of the healthcare system often sabotage well-being. As medical conditions become neglected, denial is an unintended detour to certainty.

Can we construct Advance Care Directives to be congruent with quality of life? There is no doubt that "right" decisions made earlier in life expand quality to later years. Ironically, retirement is considered the golden years—most people believe the best years occur during midlife. Do we make the most of the best years or anticipate the best is yet to come? Being conscious of this deadline, attention should be given to the preamble's connection to the pursuit of happiness. In prefacing the golden years with this initiative, we avert the scramble to find happiness as life nears its end.

Naturally, a preamble to Advance Care Directives precedes its commencement and is usually deferred until we confront life-threatening illness. We tend to wait and determine whether life-sustaining measures seem worthwhile. Serious illness compels us to beat the odds and sustain life. In good health, we take for granted the ability to determine the courses of action. When faced with serious illness we tend to follow physicians' directions. Negating the thinking necessary to preambles concedes leadership to a wait-and-see approach. Elderly people with good intentions and limited choices suffer poor outcomes. Despite taking charge, time does not heal all. Nevertheless, dignity prevails by remaining in front of the situation.

WISH 14:

Co-Establish Consternation with Constitution

Procrastination is the bane of certainty, sabotaging dignity. Disaster preparedness safeguards and promotes dignity as the forefront to the constitution of Advance Care Directives. Companies and organizations commence from a good idea. Their preamble or mission statement is a declaration and reason for the purpose and principles of the institution. Aside from doing everything possible to make this institution succeed or sustain itself, the larger ideal of Advance Care Directives is to establish a fundamental purpose and guiding principles that provide peace of mind through moral standards. The more certainty is ingrained in our preamble, the less peril we endure at the end of life, or when a company fails.

Notably, the Preamble to the U.S. Constitution lists stirring ideals and truths that honor the need for a preamble for an Advance Care Directive. The Constitution inspires self-governance as the path to freedom. This path extracts the certainty of being right from our founding fathers:

> *We the People of the United States, in Order to form a more perfect Union, establish Justice, insure domestic Tranquility, provide for the common defense, promote the general Welfare, and secure the Blessings of Liberty to ourselves and our Posterity, do ordain and establish this* [Advance Care Directive].

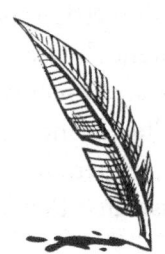

The concept of forming a more perfect union between life and death during midlife becomes possible through Advance Care Directives. With justice served and established, certainty rings true and ensures domestic tranquility. Healthcare plans provide for the common defense against illness and promote general welfare. To secure the blessings of liberty for ourselves and posterity we need Advance Care Directives that free us from overindulging in life-sustaining measures, over-treating and over-medicating natural diseases. The totality of every person becomes blessed by the liberty realized through death.

Taking stock of life and a personal constitution acknowledges needing to die and having ups not to die, including things we cannot change and things we can. When domestic tranquility is appreciated by having a doctor in the house, I encourage people to earn their own medical degree, particularly in their own area of personal illness. Ensuring domestic tranquility is realized through self-educating rather than praying away disease. "And where did you get your medical degree?" is often interpreted as a derogatory question. This "medical degree" is conferred through the wisdom of the well-known Serenity Prayer:

> *God, grant me the serenity to accept the things I cannot change;*
> *the courage to change the things I can;*
> *and wisdom to know the difference.*

My wisdom to know the difference comes from caring for thousands of patients who view their health in different ways, realizing that one size does not fit all. What is disabling to one patient empowers the next. The worst-case scenario for one is the best opportunity for another. How we react toward terminal illness makes all the difference in the world. It takes courage to recognize the things we can change. Each of us has the innate capacity for wisdom and domestic tranquility, but negates how to use these to our advantage, potentially leaving us incapacitated.

The very premise of Advance Care Directives acknowledges the possibilities of being both incapacitated and self-determined. Advance Care Directives with preamble considerations envision more certainty than incapacitation as worry dissipated through tranquility. Typically,

Advance Care Directives defer that tranquility, giving special deference to what doctors deem to be the right course of action. Advance Care Directives with a preamble highlight the notion that tranquility begins with self-governing.

The preamble provides the necessary guidelines to govern distressing situations. Self-governing applies personalized choices that promote an individual's preferred quality of life. Advance Care Directives with preambles give forethought to being sick enough to die when the situation arises. It's natural to lose our surefootedness while advancing closer to the edge of death. A directive to sustain life seems admirable, but life is tenuous. It can leave patients on unsteady ground. Convinced that we are not supposed to have cancer or heart disease, we linger in opposition to having these diagnosed, and rarely acknowledge that people die of these afflictions. Some of the worst patients I encounter are those steeped in the futility and misery of denial. Misery loves company and becomes contagious.

While an older woman detailed her medical complaints, I caught her daughter glaring up from the book she was reading. Her eyes conveyed that it was time for her mother to die if life was so miserable. With complaints of age, illnesses, medications and living situations, decisions made to retreat from life confront the lengths patients may take in order to perpetuate misery. When misery means we are not in it to win it, the mind might wish to know it from the beginning. Hold a forum and formulate a preamble.

WISH 15:

Co-Ordinate Flexibility with Rigor Mortis

Our personal level of fitness impacts our ability to deal with illness. Beyond having a strong mind and body, we need to maintain flexibility. Having a strong-willed and obstinate nature works against resiliency. Similar to Advance Care Directives, fitness plans are geared toward going the distance until we are tapped out. Regimens that allow for flexibility provide the added benefit of being able to *pause, center and shift*; take a breath, reevaluate, and reinvigorate. Elderly people who exercise routinely are quite limber. The mental and emotional flexibility to give and take is a necessary component for Advance Care Directives, providing the ability to end life gracefully.

Age creeps up slowly until suddenly, we cannot touch our toes. Stretching is the wellspring of youth. Not only does stretching create space in a degenerative spine, it can inspire a person to dig deeper, reach further and become aware of those areas in life that still are resistant. My preamble peers at the horizon with the need to be physically, mentally and spiritually elastic and shock resistant.

Many patients visiting the Emergency Department say, "I've done all I can." When asked if they have stretched that day, typically, the answer is "no" followed by the realization of needing to do more. The certainty of being right is fueled by the need to stretch. Naturally, we feel better after stretching, enabling us to live life more fully. Sadly, it seems difficult to find time to exercise and too easy to become set in our ways. The time to fight for wellness is early in life, not at the end of life.

Life becomes riddled with aches, pains and remorse through cultivating a wait-and-see attitude and we soon discover exactly why unhealthy habits impact health negatively. One elderly gentleman was diagnosed with lung cancer after 25 years of smoking. His death sentence was predicted to be anywhere between nine months to nine years. It was difficult it was for him to move on the stretcher, suggesting his quality of life was compromised by this lack of flexibility. When life feels compromised, I might plead for a shorter death sentence.

A preamble takes necessary steps to face challenges in life with courage and resolve. In addition, a preamble provides inroads to managing an existing debilitative state like, for example, chronic back pain. Some people deny being able to manage their back pain through being sedentary, overweight or excessive suffering. "What are you doing to stretch the muscles around the spine that support your back?" Such a question may raise considerations about strengthening the core in support of the spine and reducing waistlines that stress the spine.

Moreover, belief systems are wrought with tension that we store in our back or hip pockets. I realize that my backbone aligns and butts up against opposing beliefs that grip and ratchet my back, shearing intervertebral discs.

Dr. Brugh Joy shared the insight that beliefs and moral conscience stem from our mothers. I picture the "divine mother" as the Statue of Liberty, holding the torch that guides moral attitudes. My mother and I agree to disagree on many issues. However, I never thought about these issues taking a toll on my back. By lacking the appreciation of how the mind affects the body, there is little regard for the mind's ability to manage pain. Successfully managing pain begins with letting go of hurtful beliefs that contribute to pain and no longer serve the person's ability to self-govern effectively.

Describing illness as "critical" underscores other factors at play. While feeling uncertain in situations, we are typically left in the dark. In my virtual black bag I carry *Anatomy of the Spirit* by Carolyn Myss. She writes, "Biography becomes biology."[5] Generally, patients' stories can be traced back to life-altering events that triggered the beginnings of their symptoms. It is fascinating to appreciate the connection. Most revealing is what people choose to do with this information. What belief system contributes to the breakdown of our capacity to deal with critical illness? How do we integrate illness into our lives once we are reminded to *pause, center and shift?*

The certainty of being right rests unconsciously on the backbone of personal security. This security originates from the protective arm of our parents and family support, giving us the confidence that someone is likely there to catch us when we fall. The preamble for Advance Care Directives forewarns of impending assaults to health and personal security, rarely expanding consciousness of abandonment. Waiting to see how personal security disintegrates is a setup for terror not dignity. When planes flew into the World Trade Center on 9/11, I no longer believed others could guarantee my personal security. By coincidence, I began to practice yoga that fall with the intention of helping my back. What emerged in the aftermath was the need to realize personal security for myself, which is imperative to dignity.

In retrospect, the concept that a healthy back begets a healthy life expands and elaborates upon the connection between a strong back and personal security. Personal security feels like being safe at home base; yoga relates to me as sitting on home plate. In the ballgame of life, I run between bases, catch high flies, miss ground balls, am hit between the eyes and/or safely slide home or get tagged out. Nevertheless, I work toward planting my sit bones onto the yoga mat of home base to regain my bearings.

The practice of yoga, like a preamble to Advance Care Directives, is where I set aside time to check out the biology of my body. This is my time to question how my body feels in the moment and observe if there is more space that could be given to expand the breadth and depth of my personal security that empowers decision-making capacity. Indeed, "I need some space to figure things out." Yoga offers that space. I sympathize with people who confront challenging life decisions without a go-to plan that allows them enough space to repeatedly *pause, center and shift*.

The practice of yoga correlates to the practice of medicine as an art. The art of medicine is appreciated through the abstract nature of illness, attempting to distinguish which pieces are conscious and which are unconscious. What is paramount to preambles is exploring the unconscious material that prevents us from letting go of life. Could digging yoga allow me to dig my own grave? Self-preservation through yoga intertwines personal security with death and dignity.

One of my yoga instructors uses the analogy that the body is like a padlock, composed of a body, shackle and locking mechanism. Typically, padlocks protect valuables—like dignity. When in a dilemma, we hope to be able to pop the shackle and break other chains that bind. Through the practice of yoga, one learns to twist and turn the ball bearings or discs in an intricate process that allows the locking mechanism to release.

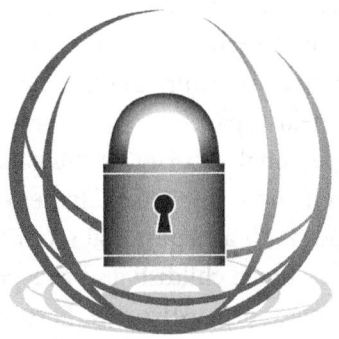

Through proper correction and body alignment, the free flow of energy within the body is experienced. This surge of energy liberates a person's being and empowers personal security. As I left class one day, I remarked to the instructor, "Everything came together again." I was secure in knowing my life was not perfect, but I left perfectly aligned, energized and open to its challenges.

Personal security often connotes hanging on to a stuffed animal, blanket, cell phone, best friend or family member. Yoga acknowledges the need for attachment along with the capacity to let go. We become perilous when there is no imperative to letting go. NPR illustrated this conflict in a Storycorps podcast titled—*With a Veteran's Life in Peril, His Parents Take up the Fight*. Erik Schei's skull was shattered by a bullet while serving in Iraq. Physicians determined that he would never be capable of caring for himself. His father remembered Erik once asked him to, "Pull the plug if anything ever happens." Erik's mother was adamant that unless he was declared brain dead, she would assume responsibility for his care and personal security. The story ends with Erik smiling every day while living in regret—repeatedly stating, "I'm sorry, Mom."

Human-interest stories often shine a light on the boundless nature of love. These stories are selfless and heartwarming demonstrations of how love maintains attachments through sickness and in health. Nevertheless, personal love becomes misconstrued with unconditional love. Brugh Joy described unconditional love as being heart-centered, impersonal, indifferent, altruistic and essentially divine. When personal security is attached to personal love and that attachment comes at our own peril. Yoga, described as "yoking with the divine," generates a connection between personal security and the inherent impersonal, unconditional love that streams from indifference circulating from the middle ground of the heart-space.

When cultivating personal security as the precursor to dignity, the preamble becomes even more important. Experiencing a midlife crisis involves a threat to both faith and personal security. During this type of crisis there is a tendency to act childish and irresponsible, suggesting we may no longer be ourselves or trustworthy. Personal security is bent on being ourselves, but sometimes wishful thinking prefers someone else take responsibility for our lives. Calamities allow faith to be reformed through these midlife experiences. Many patients place more faith in family members during times of crisis than in themselves. Our preamble establishes whether we assume more or less personal responsibility.

St. Luke's message: "Physician, heal thyself" is a proverbial call to action to practice what I preach. Patients rarely expect to heal themselves until encouraged by others or discover it from within. Personal security allows an individual to be a do-it-yourselfer. Preambles generate awareness that there is no personal security when choosing to live in denial of life's abundant resources. However, most patients insist, "I don't know what to do." Lacking the awareness of creating our own realities and destinies leaves most of us helpless. Predestination does not provide an exact hour of death; however, we all understand death to be on the horizon.

Some people create more uncertainty through procrastination, expecting that serious illness is best understood and managed by the experts. Dignity provides a person with the ability to take all the credit and responsibility for their own destiny. Creating a plan with identifiable objectives and goals protects my dignity. Having a well-thought-out preamble for Advance Care Directives overrides the tendency to procrastinate and predetermines the allocation of assets. In the marriage between life and death a prenuptial agreement is necessary to determine which assets are deemed to be truly personal keepsakes.

We are encouraged through family planning to be responsible in regard to the creation of life based on religious beliefs and personal preferences. Advance care planning applies similar moral consideration. We broach difficult conversations about prolonging or ending life as prompted by Advance Care Directives. Whatever actions are considered, spiritual and moral overtones enter into the decision-making process. I view my body as the temple and temporary dwelling for my spirit. The spirit can transcend the body at any moment, suggesting the need to release mortal attachments at a moment's notice. When the body-spirit connection is forsaken, the advance care preamble and prenup provide grounds for divorce.

Patients arriving in the ED either walk erect or are hunched over, in a wheelchair or strapped onto a gurney. Ambulatory patients maintain an easy confident pace or appear hurried, anxious, embarrassed or belligerent. ED personnel may not know the patient's particular medical complaint, but body language provides some idea of how the patient is equipped to handle the situation. Any field trip to the ED mortuary of mortality provides this trial run for exploring how we deal with death's inevitability. Most people dread being in the ED, since it easily symbolizes the gateway to death.

Preparation is required to deal with the inherent stress of higher education. The preamble for advance care planning includes educating ourselves about the serious medical condition being confronted. Preparation is invaluable and necessary; procrastination only creates more uncertainty. During preparation, we can opt to modify our belief system through proper channels of listening. By educating ourselves and asking questions, we begin to listen for guidance that supports certainty.

WISH 16:

Co-Opt Close-Mindedness with Listening

There are days spent in the Emergency Department when every medical complaint has a definitive diagnosis and patient satisfaction soars. On other days, nothing makes sense and patients act out; the full moon is rising and the sky is falling. One difficult day, I was stunned to have the whole premise of my book was challenged. An elderly man with difficulty breathing arrived in the ED. He was angry because his doctor had told him he would never get better. This patient exclaimed, "What type of doctor tells a patient that he is going to die?" I had no response. In the same breath he insisted, "I cannot live this way any longer."

As I stood dumfounded, I reminded myself that the customer is always right and chose not to disagree. What type of doctor provides the certainty of death to patients and what type of doctor offers a tedious wait-and-see approach? Occasionally, patients use the physician as a punching bag, so physicians bob and weave between telling patients what they want to say and what the patient wants to hear. Some patients do not wish to know that a particular illness will kill them, while others prefer to know the end is near. Knowledge is power and knowing the end is near provides control and closure. When knowing that prolonging life is not advantageous, opting for resolutions over options connects the certainty of being right with making wise decisions.

Every step during the process of dying presents an opportunity to become centered in certainty through mindful listening. While patients' intentions are to listen carefully to the doctor, they are also engaged in an internal dialogue that creates a necessary distraction that guards patients from having to really understand what their illness means. The most effective listeners know that what is unspoken can be more enlightening than what is being communicated verbally. The auditory nerve connected to the brain needs the audacity to remain unobstructed in order for synapses to connect understanding and truth with certainty and rightfulness.

Denial, the initial stage of coping, greatly compromises the ability to listen. We may only hear what we wish to hear and lose appreciation of the bigger picture. When closing our ears to the prospect of death we negate the presence of mind to address its perplexities. By tuning out, we become vulnerable, gullible and avoid discussions that likely make us responsible for our own deaths. Therefore, hospice care is rarely open for consideration by people who prefer not to hear they are dying. Preambles provide the thinking that rescinds denial, making room for dignity.

Denial is reversed into an overreaction when patients without a serious illness are convinced they have a looming life-threatening illness. When defenses intensify, physician/patient communication reaches an impasse. Do patients prefer a doctor to respect their denial or provide them with an honest professional opinion? It takes a good patient to be a good doctor. Over time, I realized that the best patient is the best listener. When certainty and dignity arrive at an impasse, we are challenged to *pause, center and shift* from resentment to being resourceful and purposeful.

By actively listening for our own personal calling in life, purpose in life unfolds. Well-defined purpose raises an appreciation of being talented, resourceful and fulfilled. Dignity becomes lost when there is no purpose to life. Many elderly patients experience this conundrum. It is difficult to look back over life and express satisfaction in having fulfilled a purpose when it was never defined. Certainty cultivates the acknowledgement and declaration of a purpose. Once declared, deliberate steps are taken to realize its full potential and then allow its actualization to dismiss extending life indefinitely.

We prepare for the end of life by having purpose in mind. Do elderly patients know their purpose in life? How can they know their lives were complete without realizing their purpose? Most view their purpose as self-perpetuating rather than self-fulfilling.

Exploring this line of thinking with my parents, my mother's response was to "do for others." My father's motto was "to live and let die." While these maxims provided great insights to the mind of each parent, I couldn't tell whether either felt they had completed their purposes in life. My father, in particular, failed to demonstrate his avowed intent to "let die." In retrospect, I should have phrased my original question more succinctly.

Clarity of purpose is achieved by completing the sentence:

I manifest _____!

My mother would likely say: *I manifest order!* She was supervisor at every job she ever held while raising seven children. Everything is either black or white in her world. If something does not fit her sense of order, it is ignored, disregarded or discarded. She believes that everything has its place and that there is a place for everything. If I appear to compartmentalize my life, this is her influence. My father continues to be challenged by my mother's expectations. She will have to bury him to fulfill her purpose of creating order. *Orderliness is next to godliness*; that's how my mother would proclaim it. I have no doubt her heavenly task will be to supervise God.

The purpose of my father is: *I manifest abundance!* Born and raised on a farm, he realized planting seeds and harvesting crops. As an adult, his seed produced a large crop of offspring from a woman who was told she was barren. With an eighth-grade education and sibling ridicule, he suffered from low self-esteem. Through perseverance he amassed a retirement benefit package far exceeding that of my college-educated mother. He is proud of his son, the doctor, being an offspring of his own intelligence. With an abundance of thanksgiving, I hope my father reaps what has been sown in the harvest that awaits him in the afterlife.

For my purpose: *I manifest wound care!* I look, listen and feel for opportunities to cleanse grit from the surface, wipe up blood spills, suture gaps, shield wounds from further assault and soothe pain. Simultaneously, I strive to heal the wounds of my own inner child through caring for others. Naturally, going deeper into wounds inflicts pain. Shards of glass and shrapnel left in wounds fester, become a boil and need to be removed. It is preferable to deal with pain in the moment rather than let it remain dormant, triggering delayed hypersensitivity.

Having a purpose in life makes us resourceful. Being resourceful provides the opportunity to cultivate strength and solace. Whom do we listen to with a grain of salt and whom do we listen to as the voice of reason? While my mother was considering whether or not my father would benefit from yet another round of physical therapy, she rolled her eyes. Dad was on his best behavior when the therapist was present; he ignored the therapist's advice after she had left. Mom listened to her children's advice and tried to figure out what was best for my father, creating a dilemma. Whose suggestions seem to offer the voice of reason?

While meandering through life, listening occurs best in the absence of distraction. If we identify the voice of reason connected to certainty, effective listening minimizes suffering. Many patients with chronic illness receive mixed messages from doctors in the ED and from specialists. These patients express frustration and finally insist on coordinated efforts, asking that everyone assemble in one room and arrive at one agreed-upon, reasonable treatment plan. Patients often want someone else to determine what plan is best for them, but then complain that their thoughts and feelings are not being heard.

WISH 17:

Co-Habitat Challenges with Centeredness

Inevitably, the duplicity of human nature creates space for us to be centered in the tension of opposites. We are pulled in many directions when deciding on the best course of action. We primarily seek evidence-based treatment, yet prefer our experience speak to the evidence. How we feel about a particular treatment may be more important than its scientific proof. This argument is heard in the recent debate concerning what ailments can be treated with medical marijuana and what ailments people prefer it be permissible. Personal insights afford us a level of preference and allowance. These insights lead to enlightened revelations.

Life presents a multitude of opportunities to be still and centered amid the tension of opposites. Yoga instructors say, "Listen to your body; where your eyes go, the body follows." Typically, we become— "crossed-eyed"—while dying—one eye focused on staying alive and the other peering at the barrel of a shotgun. Figuratively, the body becomes twisted in knots, not knowing which eye to follow. Swept up in the uncertainty surrounding death, a person's eyes are easily diverted from the center. We tend to shield our eyes from death rather than address it directly. Often dignity is duped by our duplicity, swaying back and forth rather than moving with purpose and balance. Grounded by the inevitability of death, the balance of dignity is maintained through an intuitive third eye.

I experience the tension of opposites in every yoga pose, particularly the courageous Warrior B pose. With legs widely extended, one bent and the other straight, feet aligned in an acute angle and arms reaching out, it embodies the inherent proverbial tug of war. I am centered between the past and future with the proposition to not lose my balance. Judy, one of my favorite yoga instructors, suggests that we do not practice yoga to perform splits, but to gain insight; not to exercise per se, but to expand awareness while continuing to lift and regain the center within each pose. We practice yoga to attempt something new, create flexibility and instill adaptability. Arising from the tension of opposites, individuals discover what feels right for them, not what is right for instructors, family members, or physicians.

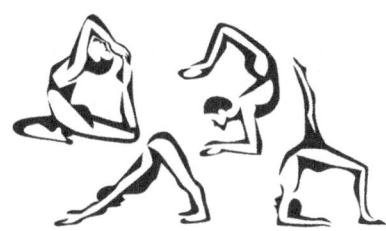

One person's center differs from that of another. We are discouraged from comparing ourselves to others while practicing yoga. The purpose of yoga is introspective; to remain focused on our own person. A connection exists between this practice and Dr. Brugh Joy's discussion regarding the heart-center having three injunctions: "Make no comparisons, make no judgments and delete the need to understand." In the practice of medicine, care providers are compelled to treat all patients the same, comparing their differences in an attempt to create more understanding. Consequently, the doctor's role becomes significant in knocking a patient off-center, negating the presence of mind given to the injunctions pumping from the heart.

Centering in the tension of opposites, we appreciate the right way, the wrong way or our way. We also become conscious of subjective personal differences between good and bad, right and wrong, life and death. The claim to" do it my way" provides the chance of a lifetime —dying with dignity intact. Strength of character continues to evolve while sitting in the tension of opposites. We gain insight as to when to act and when to let go, when to step back from the ledge or take a leap of faith. Metaphorically, this tension of opposites is the stew that simmers in a hope-filled pot of contentment. Seasoning it with compassion and lowering the heat prevents the stew from reaching a boiling point.

While stirring this stew of conflict during the period of a contemplative preamble, we might occasionally sip and indulge in a spoonful of the heart's attribute, *compassion.*

WISH 18:

Co-Conspire Empathy, Euthanasia and Exceptionalism

An understanding of true compassion allows for free will and personal choice. Many patients claim they have limited choices near the end, but claiming compassion as their choice is always available. My preamble seeks to cultivate compassion for myself and offer this same opportunity for compassion to others. Compassion seeks more understanding regarding the inner conspiracies of empathy, euthanasia and exceptionalism. A preamble views each of these subjects through the windowpane of choice.

Empathy is defined as the capacity to truly understand other's situations, emotions and motivations. Family likes to be synonymous with empathy; translating into some insistence that implies, "I know better than the patient." While dying, family members attempt to fill our shoes and step into our roles. Naturally, family members relate to each other like no one else. As they assume our responsibilities and choices, our wishes can become co-opted. Caretakers consumed by our care tend to assume our identities and may gain a sense of well-being, purpose, and personal satisfaction through the paradox of loving themselves through loving another.

With difficult medical conditions, the *caregiver* becomes the undisputed *caretaker* of identity and dignity. Doctors understand this dynamic both professionally and personally and gain satisfaction in their role as caregiver. Healing my own wounds through healing patients provides its own personal rewards. My identity as doctor is not significantly different than another's identity as mother, father, family member or close friend. Dying patients experience the loss of self-esteem, while caregivers reap the benefits of self-love through loving another. The repercussions of empathy likely foster self-love for caregivers and enhance self-pain for patients. This self-pain often manifests as both identity theft and alienation of dignity.

Restricted in the arms of a caregiver's love, patients can be tempted to relinquish control of the situation. It does not matter if the caregiver is a significant other, doctor or deity. Uncertainty within end-of-life situations will likely defer patients' wishes to the caregiver's beliefs and directives. The underlying tension in this perceived love/hate relationship between patients and caregivers mirrors the inherent love/hate conflict existing between patients and their own personal responsibilities. When left to the kindness of others, it is difficult to find peace within ourselves. Self-significance is important to end of life, yet it is often challenged when dignity is outsourced to those who embrace our suffering. Dignity is presumed when love exists under the pretext of empathy.

At its root, the definition of empathy is the ability to *embrace suffering*. To embrace another's suffering becomes addictive—because caring for others reflects marvelously upon our embodiment of love. Empathy allows us to experience and relish increased self-love while caring for others. The film *Amour*, poignantly depicts the tender, loving venture of an elderly couple before and after the wife suffers a stroke. In the aftermath, she was adamant that her husband promise to never return her to the hospital. This places the burden of her care squarely, intimately and physically on his shoulders. Transferring her back and forth between wheelchair, sofa, bed, toilet and bath becomes an awkward shuffle-step, dance and quagmire.

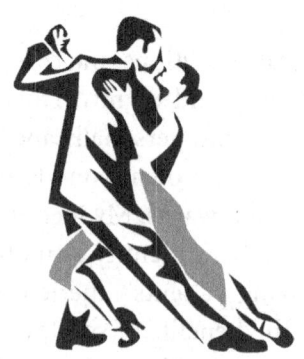

Empathy does not allow for much separation between people. With the gravity of this situation pulling the couple apart, a shaky conflict occurred in each embrace. As this woman was being held in her husband's arms, I felt a haunting willingness and uneasiness. Rewinding these dances in slow motion, I was sympathetic to the husband's challenges. With his wife's inability to speak, he attempted to read her mind and appease her needs. Her non-verbal communication was quite revealing. I sensed her body language proclaimed loudly, "Don't embrace my suffering; lift my dignity." When caregivers hold us tightly we risk certainty being squeezed from us. Trust is earned through love, but could he trust letting go of her to allow her dignity to be untethered naturally?

There is a fine line in embracing another's suffering as our own when two people are in an intimate relationship. The golden rule is a reminder to "Do unto others as you would have them do unto you." The elderly husband in *Amour* was willing to do absolutely anything and everything for his beloved wife. Their relationship was so close, he left little room for her to expire. He did not consider withdrawing any of her care and nourishment, literally, force-feeding her. Her response was to spit food back in his face and reject his love and pity. With an eventual change of heart and about face, he used her pillow to smother her suffering, end her life and lift her spirit. It is left to the viewer to determine whether the suffocation was an act of violence or benevolence.

The purpose of the wife's life had been fulfilled. As evidenced by one of her piano students performing on a global stage, she might state, *I manifest music appreciation!* Following her stroke, the wife's quality of life was such that she could no longer attend concerts. Her certainty of being right was leaving this existence when the music faded.

The film provides a valuable glimpse into real-life situations, illustrating how shame is mirrored and mired by others caring for our afflictions through codependency. The counterargument to the vice of shame is to engage shame as co-adviser, not a codependent. Shame straps us down; ideally, it can push us to pull ourselves up by our own bootstraps. The narrowness of the bootstrap reflects the narrow mindedness that creeps into conversations regarding the virtue of shame.

During the movie, the self-righteous daughter appears out of nowhere and proposes that her father take her mother's condition more seriously. He should ignore his wife's wishes and have her admitted to a care facility for proper treatment. Torn between the two most important women in his life, the husband's certainty erupts in telling the daughter to mind her own business with a virtual "shame on you" for her insolence. Simultaneously, he appears to realize his own shame in minding his wife's business by sustaining her life.

In real life, another "insolent daughter" transported her mother to the ED while her father was out of town. This woman was debilitated from a bladder infection and dehydration and her daughter insisted that her mother be placed in a nursing home. With crossed eyes, I admitted her mother to the hospital and obtained a social service consult. Patients may not always receive the best care at home, but I would welcome the comforts of home over the best care in a nursing home. Healthcare facilities are legally mandated by regulations that are imposed on patients. When I can no longer live semi-independently, I want license to become dehydrated, infected and die in my sleep. Rather than receiving the "best" care, dignity cites the best way out.

There is ample room for tension when wishes are not documented and compassion is ill defined in Advance Care Directives. Patients are not usually allowed to refuse medications or treatments in a cause to die naturally, passively and in the comfort of their own home. Compassion allows people choices; however, euthanasia is not one of the choices listed in Advance Care Directives. Generally, euthanasia is considered immoral and illegal. However, similar to recreational drug use, people sometimes use drugs as a means to escape or end their lives.

Euthanasia has become another bad word—only appropriately provided to animals. However, end-of-life conversations with patients or family members cannot occur without some consideration and tension given to prospectively or inadvertently raising concerns regarding euthanasia being enacted. Most people wish for pain and suffering to be treated but not to the point where someone stops breathing. In a very public example, Michael Jackson's early death from the administration of anesthetics and sedatives was viewed as an immoral crime. His self-determination in having these drugs be given liberally conflicted with cautionary measures of restricting these drugs. A preamble for Advance Care Directives needs to weigh in on this choice. Just as Brittany Maynard publicly declared her choice for euthanasia under the guise of "death with dignity," we may be called to cast this deciding vote for ourselves.

When parents sweat the small stuff—whether to give their child a judicious dose of Benadryl prior to a scary flight—actually dispensing sedatives to comfort and hasten the end of life for loved ones becomes even more anguishing for them as caregivers.

If there is a fine line between certainty and uncertainty, there is arguably a finer line between what is and what is not considered euthanasia. This is a highly charged word and hot topic, frequently avoided and censured. The last thing most people want on their permanent records of Advance Care Directives is *Thou shalt kill* as it could ensure their final damnation. So they agree to suffer for a period of time near the end of life rather than to risk their salvation for all eternity. The preamble for Advance Care Directives decides which of God's commandments is to take precedence. Centering in the tension of opposites, we weigh *Thou shalt love* against *Thou shalt not kill*.

The command *Thou shalt not kill* has the potential to keep patients and family members adverse to what some consider the "killing fields" of hospice. *Thou shalt love* commands and invites the guardian angels of hospice that guard and guide the transition from life to death. *Thou shalt love* permits tough love when the going gets rough, while *Thou shalt not kill* permits killing in matters of self-defense. Self-defense confronts the compassionate choice between saving life and sparing dignity. *Thou shalt not kill* implies no choice whatsoever regarding the taking of another's life. *Thou shalt love* commands upholding individual dignity. Which command distinguishes the understanding given for euthanasia?

In medical dogma, euthanasia is *the act or practice of ending life for an individual who is suffering from terminal illness or an incurable condition by lethal injection or the suspension of extraordinary medical treatment*. In layman's terms, euthanasia is referred to as "mercy killing." The inherent distress about "mercy killing" could be resolved in breaking down the term into its active and passive components. Active euthanasia occurs by *lethal injection*—perhaps the "killing" aspect. Passive euthanasia allows people to live and let die through the *suspension of extraordinary medical treatment*, affording "mercy." We provide dignity to people through mercy. However, when mercy leads to death, we opt for a hands-off approach. The conflict with euthanasia is reflected in the words of Mohandas Gandhi: "Man lives freely only by his readiness to die, if need be, at the hands of his brother, never by killing him."

Rather than insisting that euthanasia be off the table in end-of-life conversations, it needs to be more of a consideration. People need a rational appreciation of euthanasia so it feels less like a hidden agenda. They can revisit the dynamics of mercy killing within the context of dignity, weaving a personal understanding of euthanasia into Advance Care Directives. On the website euthanasia.com, I came upon on a backdoor definition of what euthanasia was not and what it could be:

> "There is no euthanasia unless the death is *intentionally* caused by what was done or not done. Thus, some medical actions that are often labeled *passive euthanasia* are no form of euthanasia, since the intention to take a life is lacking. These acts include not commencing treatment that would not provide a benefit to the patient, withdrawing treatment that has been shown to be ineffective, too burdensome or is unwanted, and the giving of high doses of painkillers that may endanger life when they have been shown to be necessary. All those are part of a good medical practice endorsed by law when they are properly carried out."

This definition of what euthanasia is *not* grants permission for passive or voluntary euthanasia when the person who dies has a will to die. Passive euthanasia emphasizes that the illness causes death, not one specific intention or action done or withheld. Many people agree that the suspension of extraordinary medical measures seems reasonable when the end is certain; however, few people consider most medical treatments above reproach. If *extraordinary* means *unimaginable* and most of us could not imagine ourselves behind the curtain of a trauma room, it is unlikely we could imagine what extraordinary measures really mean. Extraordinary means having the potential do harm as an act of violence; passive euthanasia reflects the intent toward nonviolence. Passive euthanasia respects peoples' wishes in being ready, willing and able to die.

The practice of ending suffering through the suspension of extraordinary means is considered merciful. When someone is resigned to dying, any measures that sustain life is extraordinary. People who aspire to live extraordinary and virtuous lives are worthy of dying with respect. The standard definition of virtuous is "conforming to moral and ethical principles." The definition can be clarified to include being authentic in one's ability to reason, defined by one's purpose that resonates from their heart. I ascribe to the emancipation proclamation of having an Affidavit for Passive Euthanasia (Will to Die) attached to my Advance Care Directive (Appendix III).

In the moral case for voluntary euthanasia, the Stanford Encyclopedia of Philosophy ascribes, *the importance (and responsibility) of individuals being able to decide autonomously whether their own lives retain sufficient quality and dignity to make life worth living.*[6] An affidavit is *a written declaration voluntarily made by a person under oath before an authorized official.* Having a voluntary and competent wish to die when I can no longer live semi-independently requires creating and filing an Affidavit for Passive Euthanasia. Presently, this document does not exist. The controversy of this type of document would create tension between my right to die and those who declare euthanasia is unacceptable, passive or otherwise. The self-righteous insist that all life is sacred and terminating life even passively is unacceptable.

When every child is considered a miracle, then every person is recognized as exceptional. Human beings perceived as being created in the image of God take for granted that notoriety and dignity is inherent to all human life. No blessed person should ever be permitted to die. The intent is always to save a life because life is precious. The central question is, why anyone would choose to be *exceptional*? There is no dignity to being exceptional. Moreover, by the laws of nature, there needs to be a polar opposite to exceptionalism. Hidden in the shadow of exceptionalism is compensatory personal shame. The unsightly shame that plagues those dying calls them to exceptionalism and to defy death.

The healthcare system promotes the perhaps-undeclared motto: *Exceptional Care, Exceptional Patients. Exceptional Care* sounds expensive, and becoming an *Exceptional Patient* suggests that someone might incur added pain and suffering. Exceptional patients perceive themselves as having exceptional problems and emergency situations. The operative challenge of being exceptional can be avoided, remaining somewhere in the middle of egocentricity and humility. As there is no peace in being exceptional, there is rarely peace in the ED until the *exceptional* patients are satisfied. At times the exceptionalism demanded of physicians compels them to be the hero, leaping over the queue of waiting patients to dote on exceptional patients first.

While centered between the extremes, there is peace. Indifference to the outcome aligns with being centered. When being exceptional, we are more inclined to dig our own grave by digging our heels into an unrealistic stance. Exceptionalism triggers retribution for injustices incurred in life. Exceptionalism encourages entitlement for more care and attention while additional coping skills are in play including denial, anger, bargaining and depression. Acceptance of death exchanges exceptionalism for humility. Humility is simply being grateful for having lived. It sets aside the need to be great. Humility accepts indifference, allowing for death to be less significant to the importance of our lives.

When approaching death, every person becomes like everyone else who puts their pants on one leg at a time. This simple act negates being exceptional. While aspiring to exceptionalism we must defy what is humanly possible through some mythical enterprise. Being exceptional is consistent with our divine nature and attributes that instill superpowers. I think most of us romanticize living a hero's journey, ready, willing and able to save humanity. Our uniqueness always sets us apart from the norm—placing us above others and even our own mortality. Superheroes are endowed with supremacy and do not die; they always save lives and survive.

One patient experienced chest pain following radiation therapy to his sternum. He had Stage IV pancreatic cancer and communicated in no uncertain terms, "I will survive!" The tenacity of his exceptionalism was almost pathological, bordering on delusional. His zeal to be at the extreme end of the spectrum was appreciated, but it may have made more sense for him to *pause, center and shift*. His chest pain was not cardiac in nature, but had to do with the tension between the radiation fighting the cancer and his heart-space remaining indifferent to survival. One intent of the heart-center is to reconcile death's inevitability with humility. The true hero rarely draws attention to being exceptional, typically remaining indifferent to the situation and centered in humility.

Advance Care Directives that view death as unacceptable tend toward exceptionalism. When life does not turn out as planned and death approaches, Advance Care Directives asserting exceptionalism seek more empathy while lacking provisions for voluntary euthanasia. Once a "Will to Die" is in place, the opportunity presents to die in peace. A peaceful death provides solace to those who survive. Certainty centers in the words of Richard Bach: "If you love someone, set them free. If they come back they're yours; if they don't they never were." The preamble to my Advance Care Directive seeks ways to be set free, listens for when illness will conquer me and allows me to surrender my life in a cause for personal freedom.

WISH 19:

Co-Elaborate Chosen over Conquered

A frail woman with a youthful glow and an inability to breathe—who had just been discharged from the hospital that morning—was wheeled through the revolving door of the ED. Her progressive pulmonary fibrosis was difficult to manage and she was becoming more helpless. In the preceding three months she had been diagnosed with small-cell lung cancer, but was quick to add that her oncologist was optimistic. Patients need to be in reasonably good shape to fight cancer. Her certainty of being right appeared unrealistic; naiveté overshadowed dignity.

Although she had stopped smoking, the lung damage could not be undone. She did not appear to be interested in a conversation regarding an endpoint to her life; nevertheless, her willingness to be placed on a ventilator was addressed. She was not interested in life support, but seem to prefer the conversation be left open-ended until it was absolutely necessary. An incessant battle was being waged between her lung disease and rationality. She focused on improving her health, while I would consider the feasibility of surrendering, given her impending demise.

"People should know when they are conquered," says a laudable, though laughable quote from the popular film *Gladiator*. I saw it advertised on a T-shirt in reference to the dominance of a football team. I wondered if the man sporting the T-shirt would have the insight to know when he was conquered or if this was strictly in reference to others. Napoleon stated, "He who fears being conquered is sure of defeat." Those not willing to contemplate defeat are certain to sabotage their dignity. Intellect vacillates we will be conquered by death and accepting the concept of being conquered with the realization that *we win some; we lose some*. Dignity allows for the acknowledgement of the loss; defeat gripes my soul.

A preamble should acknowledge that all steps and roads lead to a final destination. Being predestined to die requires a watchful eye for when the wagons begin to circle. Watchful waiting perceives and accepts the idea of being *chosen* or *complete* rather than being *conquered*, making end-of-life conversations more palatable.

Typically, being *conquered* requires waging war in a fight to the bitter end. Being *chosen* is an invitation to transcend life after crossing the finish line. Feeling energized by the effort to live and not die, the need to fight to the bitter end will leave us massacred. As the wagons circle, ill-fated patients confront illness as the enemy forcing them to surrender. Living in opposition to being conquered by death, patients become careless about whose feelings are sacrificed in battle. How much are others enlisted in our own personal battles? Apt to sweat as the wagons begin to circle, patients are encouraged to *do no harm* to self and others. In being chosen, there is a call to *choose this, not that* as an act of empowerment over annihilation.

Not knowing what to do at the end of life is actually much more about not recognizing when we become conquered. By remaining in the dark and denying the end, we are likely to be subjected to the massacres or bloodbaths of intensive care treatment. When succumbing to a particular illness would we encourage healthcare providers to still give us all they can? Caring staff find it extremely difficult to act as "yes" people for futile patients saying "no" to being conquered. When planning an exit strategy, do we resign to feel complete or expire from a position of resistance? The preamble begins to realize our greatest weakness as our greatest strength.

Choosing to exit sooner rather than later ensures we do not overstay our welcome. A pre-planned peaceful exit from treatment implies the wisdom to advance cautiously, avoiding the onslaught of unnecessary treatment. The goal in driving the treatment plan is not to be hauled off the road by EMS, ending up in the ED. Ideally, there would be signs along the way: "Proceed with Caution" or "Exit Here." By attempting to outlast a terminal illness, we can easily run out of fuel and lack the energy necessary to steer conversations regarding the end of life. Requiring roadside assistance has the consequence of being towed or perhaps told what to do. When the going gets tough, the tough maintain the feeling and certainty of having reached their final destination.

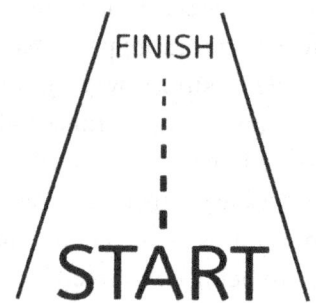

Even as the body may be decomposing from disease or injury, most people are not programmed to accept being conquered. A quadriplegic veteran who was vehemently opposed to receiving bedside assistance until it was too late arrived in the ED. Despite his refreshing free spirit, the staff literally got wind of his rotting flesh. I was mortified when we discovered his incontinence was related to a bedsore that had eroded into his bladder. His strong willpower ignored his body's decay. His insurance company had previously recommended hospice given his end-stage medical condition. He was indignant that no one wished to touch him much less heal him. Being conquered is what happens when we lack the strength to care for ourselves.

The mind is geared toward reaching milestones in self-sufficiency and achievement, but the body is apt to become weak. One of my mother's favorite terms of encouragement is, "If at first you don't succeed, try, try again." However, there comes a point in waxing and waning when we risk overcompensating. Our culture is heavily focused on anti-aging, but people need to accept the reality that if they live long enough they will eventually age and die. They will likely become sick and tired and old. Only the healthy die young.

People need to know when they have been conquered. Similarly, alcoholics ought to know when they have had one too many, children ought to know obedience, physicians ought to know what they are doing and

God ought to never abandon the faithful. Critical thinking reminds us to exchange *ought* for certainty. Sadly, many people who were emotionally conquered early in life are no longer open to being coached. As they become fixed in their ways, they are less likely to remain open to possibilities and change. Stubbornness undermines the ability to be coaxed and coached. Accepting the offer to rise above closed-mindedness allows dignity to guide a person and inspire certainty.

To gain completeness, on has to acknowledge that there is a time to live and a time to die. Completeness does not concede defeat. Are there particular situations in which we would readily declare being conquered, granting ourselves permission to die? When activities of daily living become a struggle, we fail a mini-stress test. If someone is no longer ambulatory, is unable to transfer independently to a wheelchair, or cannot wipe their butts, independence is long gone. We all recognize this, but Advance Care Directives are typically vague as to when loss of independence leads to surrender. Once conquered, I would choose comfort care and greatly minimize accessing acute care.

It is emotionally uncomfortable for physicians to tell patients they are dying. The patient benefits from reading between the lines while discussing terminal illness. As the wagons circle, few people wish to hear they are doomed. It is more comfortable for physicians to distract patients with offers of treatment rather than a respectable exit strategy. Distraction supports an ongoing state of denial; fueling unrealistic hopes with potentially devastating effects for all. When patients lack the perception that terminal illness culminates in death, I remember my mother's old saying, "You're going to be late for your own funeral."

Ignoring death creates confusion, confrontation and controversy. People have a tendency say one thing and do another. The level of support required for people at the end of life is anyone's guess. Patients may be informed that there is no cure, but varying treatments are suggested. This gives patients mixed messages—are they to face death or hope for survival? Most treatments at the end of life are palliative, perhaps prolonging despair. When vulnerable patients outline their plan, it can challenge other doctor to wonder who is advising them. Who takes away patients' dignity and creates delusional thinking?

Offering hope to terminally ill patients and family members needs to be balanced with providing certainty to dying with dignity. When the die is cast, do we face the end with courage? I have become bolder in directly stating to patients, "You are going to die from this illness." However, patients frequently are attentive to what they prefer to hear. Being uncomfortable with the concept of being chosen to die, "Do what you need to do to keep me alive," is frequently the statement that overrides any plan for surrender. Many doctors tend to oblige this and concede that under their watch, surrender and death are not options.

Doctors rarely choose to be fatalistic as this equates to us as being failures. When a doctor tells patients they are dying, patients will look for someone else to tell them what they wish to hear. The path to dignity easily becomes diverted by acquiescing to life-sustaining measures. Physicians are not always as forthright with information that relays bad news with certainty. This often delays the patient's realization of having crossed the finish line despite having reached the dubious end zone. Without a clear finish line established, patients are easily left feeling incomplete at the end of life. Physicians who do provide patients the certainty of a finish line allow them the experience of a peaceful surrender amid the simultaneous surge of relief and self-fulfillment upon crossing it.

People often ask friends to tell them when they are *too far gone*. "If I ever get that crazy, will you let me know?" Patients' caregivers are often apt to be more polite than bold, rarely confronting a patient's misperceptions. Some people prefer downplaying memory lapses and physical or emotional disability. The elderly circumvent answering questions, hoping that others will not notice their mental slipping and sliding. When patients or caregivers do not acknowledge that life has a finale, the disconnection easily leads to unrealistic thinking. However, these disturbing situations warrant attention.

Illness prevents us from realizing our best, but will it serve with regards to being chosen and with the search to find the best way out of its entrapment? Many patients consider themselves done when their health issues outweigh the benefits of living. When the pros and cons of daily activity are curtailed by severe pain and suffering, many disabilities are not compatible with enjoying life. When decompensation results from illness that has little chance for recovery, it may be time to consider how greed potentially contributes to hoarding life and hanging on by life support.

When life expectancy is exceeded, the medical examiner typically releases the deceased without further investigation. The assumption is that this person lived a full life and died of natural causes. Despite remaining active and having the energy of a locomotive, travel insurance is not underwritten for someone expected to die at any time. While living on borrowed time, anything can happen. Normally, the aging process catches people off guard as they remain in denial that life will end. More expectancy and disappointment arises out of this denial. When life expectancy is exceeded, careful consideration needs to be given to treating ourselves with mercy rather than interventions that disrespect the natural course of an illness.

Life comes at us fast, but dying seems like an eternity when faced with terminal illness. Despite implementing treatment, the possibility of losing the battle may still need to be acknowledged. Some people appear shocked that terminal illness causes death, particularly when they have fought against an illness for an extended duration. It is in a patient's best interest to know when to surrender. The irrational belief of actually conquering terminal illness directly challenges certainty and dignity. When disallowing surrender and assuming a greater stance against defeat, we sacrifice the courage to embrace being chosen to die.

WISH 20:

Co-Join End-Stage with Predetermination

"End-stage" anything—cancer, COPD, heart disease, liver disease or kidney disease—creates the awareness that illness has a finale. The virtual wagons that are circling suggest impending doom. As the finale approaches, patients need to reconsider any thoughts about expending energy on paddling upstream. Their final days can be spent in better ways. Accepting end-stage reality allows the disease to have one last round or flare-up and then use it as the last hurrah. Dignity is usurped by Einstein's definition of insanity: "Doing the same thing over and over again and expecting different [quality of life] results."

Sometimes the message suggesting we are conquered might be seen on the first wagon that displays the sign, "Not a Surgical Candidate." People like the idea of avoiding surgery, but like the idea of expeditiously removing a tumor or correcting a medical condition. However, to be labeled as not fit for surgery suggests there are serious underlying medical problems. The next stage of debilitation follows the second wagon parading the sign, "Medical Treatment Only." Any limitation to my care suggests my choices are being compromised. It follows that if my independence is drastically diminished, I prefer the next wagon to read, "Comfort Measures Only."

"Comfort Measures Only" has different meanings. Personally, I define comfort measures as provisions that ease transition from this life. Physicians' abilities to provide comfort is better understood and granted when patients freely express being completely finished. Once a patient is ready to have life end, physicians need to proceed with more of a hands-off approach while maximizing comfort. Once this happens, life becomes less stressful. The pathology and progression of an illness provides direction to the preamble's prospect of a peaceful ending.

Many agree that being kept alive by a machine is unacceptable; yet, there are hospitals largely dedicated to caring for ventilator-dependent patients. While dependent on machines in order to breathe, these patients are one power failure away from being conquered. When checking the settings on patients' ventilators, it prompts thoughts regarding patients having their own parameters for then the machine is to be disconnected? Utilizing ventilator support is a sensible option for patients expected to recover, but may be unwise for terminal patients suffering from respiratory failure due to COPD, ALS, congestive heart failure or cancer. Addressing life support with the wife of an Alzheimer's patient became awkward when she mentioned that he would refuse it if he were to become a "mindless vegetable." Despite her understanding of his wishes, she remained open to having him placed on a ventilator if needed.

With respect to the survival rule of three—when three organ systems have failed—I feel the patient has endured enough. In a car accident, the automobile does not need to be completely damaged for the insurance company to consider it totaled; extensive repair is considered cost-prohibitive. A patient suffering with terminal illness might reach the stage of being considered totaled. It seems more humane than expecting the person to keep driving until collapsing. The idea of a brand new car or a brand new life is exceedingly more attractive to most.

If there is ever a sign that health is headed in the wrong direction, particularly during the aging process, we need only look for answers below the waist. One of the more humiliating situations in life is experiencing the total loss of bladder or bowel control. When it relates to a procedure or seizure, we recover from the humiliation. If the situation progresses to becoming reliant on product like Depends, we might look at the diaper-like garment as a sign of not only being child-like, but conquered. It is not uncommon for people to dream about being in a public place dressed only in their underwear. The real nightmare is waking up to the reality of someone needing to change our diaper.

Similar to the view being obstructed below the waist and people not knowing they are conquered is the notion that waist size does not matter. How much yardage in life is lost when inches are gained? People may not know they are conquered while obese. I clue into this when patients fail to mention obesity being one of their medical problems. Health-care professional often feel defeated addressing health issues when dis-cussions about weight loss are a nonstarter. During the mindset of a preamble, consideration might be given to connecting the certainty of being right with willpower. Lack of willpower is a measure of weakness and sabotages self-esteem and well-being. The certainty of being right seemingly supports the certainty of being right with body weight.

Another clue that the wagons are circling may be realized by what seems to have surrendered below the waist. The loss of libido and sexual function has inherent psychosocial implications. Sex is one of the ways we "score" in the game of life; impotence connotes failure. An individu-al's inability to engage in sex could easily affect his or her desire to live. Regardless of the cause, impotence diminishes procreative forces and might subconsciously affect a deeper level of engagement with others. With libido considered to be an inherent life force, speculation could be given as to how effective CPR would be while trying to resuscitate the heart.

Similar to the loss of libido is the loss of appetite. Many people rec-ognize that when animals stop eating, the end is probably near. Many elderly and terminally ill patients are unwittingly brought into the Emergency Department by family members hoping to restore their appetites and receive hydration. In addition, I care for nursing home patients who repeatedly remove their feeding tubes. Is the tube pulled out consciously or by accident? When the sustenance of life no longer holds appeal, by whose order are we to be force-fed? What other types of medical interventions are deemed necessary when patients no longer wish to eat? As the wagons circle, do we prefer they be stocked with supplies to keep us alive?

Many in healthcare feel a sense of defeat when looking over a lengthy list of prescribed medication. Normally, the longer the list suggests the lessened possibility of a healthy life. My impression is that patients are conquered when they lack awareness of their prescribed medication and purpose. Is there ever an intention to limit the amount of medi-cation necessary to achieve quality of life? Is there a choice to defer medications that equate to feeling "medicated" as being conquered? The certainty of being right aspires to avert being kept alive as some type of biochemistry experiment. We assert our right to be human by withdrawing medications that no longer support the ability to feel or die naturally.

Family forces amid circling wagons sound the call to arms, seeking answers as to why loved ones are deteriorating while clearly dying. This absurdity eludes the weak patient, but is nonetheless serious to family members. Growing tired of living is apparent in the elderly. While engaging in the fight against the forces of nature, is this fight determined and respected as personal? When expected to die, failing to thrive submits a resignation to illness with a readiness to die. When caring for these patients, I wish to respect their obvious detachment from life.

Depression is a by-product of losing the battle and manifests as an anti-social personality. Many people seem to think depression is not an acceptable part of dying. Naturally, there are attempts to cheer people up who are overwrought as the wagons circle closer. I encounter the same type of cheerleading while being browbeaten at work, being told I need to smile more. Over-comforting can distract patients from expressing their true feelings. Clouding this process with a smile may result in supporting denial rather than dignity. Depression serves appropriately to weaken defenses while simultaneously releasing attachments to life. When the mind shuts out, can the shutters be pulled to shut out the world?

When a friend was diagnosed with Multiple Myeloma, life as he knew it came to an end and he considered taking his own life. Acknowledging the wish to end life equates with the knowledge of being conquered. Suicide aligns my being within the crosshairs of what makes my life worth living. While not necessarily being an advocate of suicide, assisted or otherwise, I would not discourage individuals from allowing suicidal thoughts to enter into the decision-making process regarding medical treatment. A "suicidal person" readily wishes to withhold or withdraw any measures that might prolong life.

Suicidal ideation causes concerns that we might be losing our minds and losing control over our lives. When the control center of the mind becomes compromised, people are labeled incompetent (conquered). Similar to impotence, incompetence might arouse concerns that life is less than worthwhile—simply going through the motions of living without purposeful or mindful engagement. The security inherent in having others control our lives might be desirable, but does this allow for dignity? Once decision-making capacity becomes null and void, I view the prospect of being conquered as the actual opportunity to su render.

When all treatment options have been exhausted, I visualize patients being conquered. Most people know when they are tired and wish for sleep. Priorities tend to change and what previously seemed important no longer matters. If someone like my mother believes there are never enough hours in the day, it follows that there are never enough years in life. The level of anxiety and activity in contemporary life significantly distracts from being centered. The certainty of being right syncs the level of exhaustion with the desire for peace. When completely exhausted, we assuredly deserve to rest in peace.

People are conquered when they can no longer handle the truth. In reality, the truth about death is hidden within care plans designed to sustain lives. More attention is paid to prolonging life than instilling and supporting patients' dignity. As tears flow from patients or family members at the end of life, this emotional breakdown may avoid the truth and rescind DNR orders. The best response to being chosen to die comes in the strength to handle the truth. Pretending that we are not supposed to die obstructs the truth that dying is inherent to humans. Dealing with the truth realistically and literally is a means to reconsider being patient about dying.

In the film, *A Few Good Men,* Jack Nicholson's character stands up in the witness box and sternly declares, "YOU CAN'T HANDLE THE TRUTH!" Loudly, this demeaning remark reverberates off the Navy courtroom walls. This statement begs us to differ and implores us to question how we will handle the truth. The clearest communication and acceptance of the truth occurs with the proposition, "May I have a hospice referral?" Truth emerges through the wisdom to know the difference between the things I cannot change and the things I can. Hospice grants serenity while offering a refuge for the time to die. Doctors who are for or against hospice referrals provide validation to patients who remain on the fence as to the likelihood of death being imminent.

Patients are not admitted to hospice care unless they only have six months to live. Requesting a hospice referral indicates an acceptance of being conquered with a willingness to move beyond entrapment to freedom. A friend, Omar, who could not handle the truth of being HIV positive, much less dying from HIV-related illness, never considered hospice care. He ended up on life support for nearly a month before his significant other dealt with Omar's own personal truth. My certainty lies in the belief that hospice supports and optimizes the ability to die with dignity.

A similar type of resistance to hospice prevents people from considering long-term care facilities. People are willing to consider burial locations but give little thought to their living arrangements that may be necessary as life transitions before internment. There is no dignity in being irresponsible and ignoring the range of possibilities regarding long-term care. How we withdraw from that care must also be considered. During the time to die, do we call hospice care to the bedside? What we don't preempt can come back to haunt us when abdicating personal responsibility. Hospice is a safe have that invites people to deepen their recognition that they are chosen to transcend life, potentially avoiding reactionary calls to 911.

Besides calling 911, a more immediate question presents: If today is the first day of the rest of my life, how do I wish to spend it? Do I raise a little hell by celebrating life or indulge in feeling miserable? Once conquered, I prefer to go out with a bang and have others enjoy the fireworks display as I depart. Maybe I will spend time at a spa and be pampered to death before meeting the great and powerful Wizard of Oz. Beyond simply receiving chrism to the forehead, I prefer the whole enchilada be greased and served up royally.

Hospice offers dying patients a more gentle form of healthcare. "He is a hospice patient" generally switches efforts to treating patients more kindly. Hospice patients are sacred as if being held in God's hands. By admitting the end is near there is an acceptance of being chosen with an awareness of it being in God's hands now. *Humble yourselves, therefore, under the mighty hand of God so that at the proper time he may exalt you* (1 Peter 5:6).

A peaceful ending begins with being open to the truth, allowing the truth to set us free with a dignified way out. When physicians insist more could be done—even as patients appear to be done—I find little regard and much less dignity being given to patients. The decision to keep fighting until the bitter end enacts misery. Most of us wish to die peacefully, but many default to doing everything disgracefully. Terminal illness warrants conclusion, not continuation. When a patient concludes that *nothing more should be done* prior to the doctor's statement that *nothing more can be done,* it allows for dignity to emerge through having done it "my way." This principle sets the stage for enacting Advance Care Directives.

The preamble to Advance Care Directives begins with facing the reality of death and ends with the supreme teacher calling out, "Time's up; pencils down, please." The time for finishing the preamble essay of what to do or how to act when tested by a life-threatening situation is now. Ready or not, the enactment of Advance Care Directives will ensue. If we have not properly prepared and predetermine the wishes that compassionately address our will to die, it is unlikely we have the ability to make rational decisions once the wagons circle. Through each step of the preamble, it becomes necessary to *pause* in the question of being conquered, *center* in the prospect of death and *shift* energy toward the enactment of Advance Care Directives.

PART IV

...

Enactment of advance care directives

WISH 21:

Pro-Life Disposition

With a pro-life disposition, illness is experienced as inconvenient to living. One day we might be well, the next morning we awake to a burning sensation in the nose and throat that feels like the start of a cold. Routines become disrupted by the need to take medication, carry tissues and see a doctor. The level of agitation about and tolerance of the cold is person-dependent. Some rush to the ED while others drink plenty of fluids, take extra Vitamin C and let the cold run its course. A pro-life disposition always aims to be healthy.

More than 20 years ago a good friend of mine named Gwen married a great guy who lifted her onto a pedestal and gifted her with two beautiful children. Their relationship grew through stride and strife. He is ten years her senior, but at the age of 60 he outpaced men half his age. He worked out consistently, was a regular at spinning classes and cast his fishing rod routinely. Ironically, the three of us went skiing when Gwen's first child was a bun in the oven; now her son has grown up to be a snowboard bum. Her family joined me on a recent ski trip to Utah—Gwen's husband struggled to keep up. He claimed he had not skied for a while and blamed the altitude. Upon returning home, he was overwhelmed by an avalanche of unexpected medical problems.

His initial diagnosis was acute kidney failure caused by Multiple Myeloma, a type of bone marrow cancer. His blood cells were overproducing cancerous myeloma proteins that were clogging his kidneys. Chemotherapy was initiated and spinning classes were soon replaced by dialysis treatments three times a week. Adding insult to injury, the heaviness experienced in his chest on and off the slopes was attributed to a blocked heart artery that required a stent. Along with the loss of weight, hair, energy and financial security, his appearance changed beyond recognition. He was infuriated by the injustice of these illnesses that infringed upon his prime of life and pro-life disposition.

Gwen and I met during my medical residency at the hospital's wellness center and we began to run together several times a week. Twenty years later we cherish a long-running friendship. I encouraged her to maintain a steady pace while attacking the uphill climb to save her husband's life. The same gut-wrenching heartache that sometimes occurs with running was with her every minute. We had always discussed anything and everything, keeping it real. When I suggested balancing out treatment plans with exit strategies, she became really angry.

"I am trying to keep my husband from dying; I cannot be concerned about his dignity." I might be writing a book, but she insisted, "We are not having this conversation." Her marriage was facing a major assault and breakdown in communication. She was uncertain as to how to deal with both the reality and the gravity of this situation. My intent was not to bury her husband, but to explore his dignity in this situation. However, the certainty of being right was weighing heavy for Gwen and her husband—balancing a pro-life disposition with the prospect of dying.

Her point of annoyance was well taken while the point of my book was taking shape through this conversation: Is it better to initiate this type of discussion before or after the diagnosis of a life-threatening illness? Do we enact Advance Care Directives from a comprehensive perspective or strictly a pro-life disposition?

Most people prefer not to think about a life-threatening illness, much less talk about it. We tend to keep this conversation relatively brief and nondescript. The idea that her healthy husband would ever consider reading a book like *Wishes To Die For* was absurd. Any considerations regarding him dying were decidedly out of bounds. Nevertheless, I remained intrigued by the coincidence of his illness happening at the same time I was devising Advance Care Directives with pre-determined endpoints. Despite being unjust, could the certainty of any illness still enact some way and certainty of being right? Do we continue to hope for the best from a pro-life disposition?

Any life-threatening illness prompts us to react, pushing aside wishes to know, declare and document when to call it quits. Most people ad-lib the enactment of Advance Care Directives with very little preparation, resulting in a plan that is sketchier than certain. Fortunately, my friend's illness responded to stem cell replacement therapy, but his remission is more likely temporary than permanent. Therefore, he is acutely aware that he could confront this cancer again along with further heart disease. Would he plan to do things differently in the future and simply maintain a pro-life disposition? Enacting a plan begins with thinking before we do, leaving as little to happenstance as possible.

Similar to a job interview, terminal illness is generally approached with self-promotion. We are certain of being an asset to the manager since our livelihoods are on the line. We may claim to be reliable, hard-working, a team player and willing to go the extra mile. We seek to persuade a boss or doctor that we are up to the task, ready and able to handle any possible situation or challenge. In return, we hope to receive a paycheck or positive performance review stating, "Your numbers look good." People naturally expect to sacrifice some quality of life for the job of living. No one ever wishes to be handed the dreaded pink slip or be called into the boss' office to hear, "You're fired!"

Terminal illness feels like receiving a termination notice. It can break self-esteem, lower their defenses, open the door to personal shame and lead to hysteria. Efforts that used to work in our favor become unappreciated and irrelevant. We make valiant attempts to demonstrate life is foolproof and necessary. Without a leg to stand on, people figuratively shake the other leg or build a crutch. I am amazed at the ingenuity displayed in society—many people with disabilities embody a pro-life disposition through perseverance and adaptation.

When terminal illness is diagnosed, the stage is set for responsiveness, determination and enactment. Do we fight back or surrender? Doing nothing is rarely an option. A couple of friends relayed the story of a man who was golfing and suddenly lost his balance and part of his vision. He went to the Mayo Clinic Hospital in Phoenix and was diagnosed with an aggressive, untreatable brain tumor. Dissatisfied, the man obtained a second opinion from Barrow Neurological Institute. Barrow's offered to remove the tumor, but told him there was no guarantee he would live beyond two months. I listened as my friends debated the personal merits of being pro-life.

When a stroke, heart attack or cancer occurs, we embark on a rollercoaster ride with its inherent ups and downs. Life undergoes a significant change from out with the old to in with the new. When the "new normal" is realized as being old or the odd one out, life plummets from the assault of being diseased, dependent and desecrated. Pro-life disposition begins to suck.

The gestation period from diagnosis to death may be similar to a woman who learns of an unexpected pregnancy. Arguably and profoundly, a woman confronts the same coping stages of denial, bargaining, anger, depression and acceptance—similar to receiving a life-altering diagnosis. With the advent of new life or bad news, I frequently hear the same question: "What am I going to do?" In an instant, we experience the power of God as Creator, having a huge responsibility in mapping out a plan. The moral compass spins wildly until the magnetic force of fear causes the pointer to rest in the direction of enactment, which is typically a pro-life disposition.

Our preamble to Advance Care Directives potentially addresses both family and end-of-life planning. Once the news of a fatal diagnosis can no longer be held at bay through denial, anger erupts. The indictment of an illness makes most of us feel sentenced and punished. This festering or nesting period provides time to *pause, center and shift*, knitting our thoughts into booties to either kick the illness or kick the bucket.

Ideally, planning for the future has to be differentiated from living in the future. Anger is less likely when we live in the moment and soften undying pro-life dispositions. Anger prompts fights and rage leads to further indignation. Illness is never a welcomed part of life—it is the inescapable threshold to the end of life that lacks a welcome mat. Fear or anger causes us to charge or flee. Running from death is futile, yet many people become fugitives in their passion to escape the Grim Reaper. Some prefer to turn themselves over to a higher authority. Upon surrendering, we lay down arms and diffuse defenses. Enacting Advance Care Directives anticipates the realization of mission accomplished and averts mission impossible.

Becoming caught up in tragedy is involuntary, similar to being strapped in the backseat of a car. At the wheel of the car is a family member driving the conversation and decision-making process. Certainty is difficult to realize when everything seems to be against a pro-life disposition and our own personal will. We rely on others to show us the way and provide expertise and optimism, keeping us in the game. I recall conversing with a patient who had reached his final hour of life. He and his wife were still deliberating life support in order to keep a scheduled follow-up appointment with the oncologist. Illness and death are involuntary; life support and follow-up visits are voluntary.

Similar to anger, terminal illness feels like unending conflict when losing control. Advance Care Directives are designed to regain control when life-threatening situations become out of hand. My Advance Care Directive is designed to maintain control of my life upon being diagnosed with terminal illness. I witness many people conveniently tucking their Advance Care Directives behind fear, rather than using them to actually enact their plan.

A good time to bring any issue to the surface is when we are angry. In *Conversations with God,* Neale Donald Walsch writes, "Anger is fear announced."[7] When anger arises from a life-threatening situation, it sets the tone and announces enactment of Advance Care Directives. Generally, anger gets us nowhere. Nevertheless, Mothers Against Drunk Drivers (MADD) exemplifies how their anger is necessarily geared toward being pro-life and preserving life.

On Death and Dying emphasizes that anger can erupt at any moment, once the dam of denial bursts. The scene is set for the part we were destined to play, conflated by the part of life we fear. Alongside this alter ego that claims to never be sick, we play the role of dutiful patient. Anger arises from the loss of control that results from illness and not feeling like ourselves. There is an irreconcilable difference between remaining healthy and the unanticipated consequence of becoming chronically ill.

People confront terminal illness from the perspective of giving everything with nothing to lose. Some patients claim, "I'm not afraid of anything," and then lose every ounce of self-respect as they live in denial of dying. Typically, patients' Advance Care Directives cautiously abide by doctors' orders. Opting out of these orders creates patient angst, caught between duty and dignity. Following doctors' advice, patients become angry when the treatment plan fails. Aggravation, humiliation and determination result in the double whammy of both the losing the battle and the certainty of being right. Certainty is regained when people enact Advance Care Directives that promote rising above fear and stressing the importance of remaining more engaged than enraged.

I support people who are reluctant to see doctors and adverse to undue medication and testing, particularly when their plate is already full of ailments. Anger is justified when questioning, "How much more do I need to take?" With repeat visits to the ED, patients fuel my anger and trigger me to question, "How much more am I expected to give?" Anger tends to force patients into becoming overzealous. Are there limits to being proactive? Quality of life ends when becoming obsessed with anger. A pro-life obsession with anger will sacrifice decision-making. Softening anger sanctions withdrawing interventions that irrationally sustain life.

Pro-life powers-that-be do not overtly support a plan to end life. Therefore, people obliged the effort to prolong life rather than enact directives that provide personal dignity and certainty. My intent is not to end life abruptly, but to be able to die naturally when recovery does not allow me to regain quality of life.

In anticipation of life-threatening illness, do we know from the outset if we prefer a no-holds-barred, only-going-so-far process or a nip-it-in-the-bud directive? This calls into question, "How well do I know myself?" My stubbornness tells me I am only going so far, and that less is more. To me, pro-life means being true to myself and my principles more so than necessarily saving my life. In weighing the options, foremost in my mind is having the personal freedom to do nothing. With limited capacity to compromise my convictions, coercion to treat terminal illness could result in a persistent agitated state.

Current laws are such that Advance Care Directives cannot be enacted until terminal illness has been diagnosed, or in other words, someone is expected to die within six months. My dignity does not rest upon defining terminal illness within a specific timeframe. It is based upon a directive that enacts certainty when quality of life ends. The new normal imposed by a chronic condition may or may not be terminal, but could easily end quality of life.

At that point, I prefer to see the proverbial light at the end of the tunnel through palliative care. Conceivably, the enactment of Advance Care Directives calls attention to end-of-life considerations. However, anticipating the enactment calls attention to how we perceive adapting to life in this moment. Are we angry with how life has unfolded or have we reached the stage of contentment? The more fulfilled we are today, the less likely anger will escalate through debilitating illness. I remain open to the prospect of going into the light peacefully rather than enacting a fight until the bitter end.

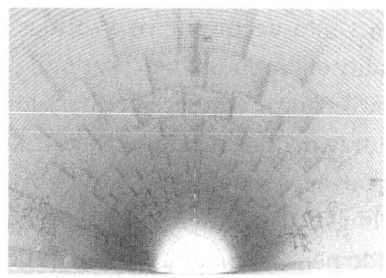

WISH 22:

Pro-Life Survival of the Fittest

A dvance Care Directives are rarely enacted from a higher purpose, but more likely from the primal fear that prompts survival of the fittest. According to author Dean Koontz in his novel *Fear Nothing,* "Illness is man's greatest predator and to a predator, fear indicates weakness."[8] Typically, illness exposes vulnerability and weakness. Becoming vulnerable to illness sparks fear, competitive ambition and separation anxiety. No one wishes to appear weak. Therefore, strength, conviction and righteousness are stoked by hope, expectation and triumph. Truly, we can never underestimate or undermine the power of "I will survive!"

As Americans, when the bomb of life-threatening illness hits, we become righteous through courageous and decisive retaliation. We adopt the Patient's Bill of Rights to every individual's right to life. As provided by the US Constitution, the pursuit of happiness permits us to pursue the inalienable right of longevity. When inalienable rights conflict with natural laws, confusion ensues between right and wrong. We are reluctant to accept any limitation to guaranteed rights and freedoms. We choose every means possible to fight for personal well-being and honor. When the threat of who we are in life conflicts with who we are while dying, we shall overcome disparity.

The array of drugs and technology in medicine rivals the armament of the US military. Healthcare providers can do either considerable damage or much good. However, understanding the mission and the endpoint is not always clear when we engage in a battle against terminal illness. Despite an abundance of resources, battles are lost and lives end. In the midst of the fight-or-flight response, adrenaline stimulates sympathetic neurons to *do or die.* If given the choice, my strategy is to allay fear with certainty, averting the rally to dial 911. I prefer not to experience my final hours behind the fetid curtain of an emergency room.

Threats to our way of life can result from acts of terror, fueling more fear, competition and provocation. In service to survival of the fittest, anger prompts rising to the occasion and fighting terror at all cost. In our darkest hours, we perceive ourselves as the dark horse unlikely to succeed. We envision ourselves to be in competition with survival. Competition sparks higher levels of achievement triggered by comparison, judgment, rivalry, and hostility. Feeling maligned sparks anger and violent outbursts. Our culture fosters competition; competition fuels violence. Anger and fear lead to further suffering and violence that disregard dignity. Cultural competition is our bloodstream but not necessarily inscribed in the Bill of Rights.

With death unacceptable, attempts to survive intensify. In the stadium of sadomasochism, pleasure is derived from the pain inflicted during football games, wrestling matches or bullfights. The thrill of brutal annihilation borders on the inhumane and grotesque, yet the transference is exhilarating. The popularity of the film *The Hunger Games* demonstrates this attraction to fight to the death. My game plan is to avoid being hurt. Depending on one's tolerance, I view suffering as both sinister and inspirational. Human beings are capable of understanding the concept of enduring suffering; animals are not. Confusingly, we often treat animals humanely and human beings inhumanely.

It is no wonder that the fear of death is more about the fear of suffering. In many cases, we face a long, drawn-out course while dying. As personal determination fades, the trilogy of family, physician and faith ignites and fires up our efforts. Passion that sustains is heartwarming, but these efforts easily become inflamed and result in inhumane treatment. I witness this fear taking over when passion flares out of control. Advance Care Directives need to act as firewalls to prevent the spread of one caregiver attempting to outdo another, causing further harm.

Love knows no bounds or impositions. Most family members rarely reconcile guilt with sitting back and doing nothing. Doing nothing appears to be uncaring, negligent and contrary to being pro-life. Yet, God help the patient whose family members' interests are wrought with competitive guilt, burdensome fear and over-compensated ego. Never mind that patients may have no appetite; they are pushed to eat one more bite and then another. The patient attempts to appease caregivers despite their illness. With the mind set on survival of the fittest, the tendency is to believe that a little more will trigger a miraculous turnabout and a second chance at life.

Certainty is never perceived as simply doing a little bit at the end of life. Certainty enacts a more definitive plan like "all or none" or "all for one." CPR is initiated because everyone deserves another shot at recovery when life has been cut short. Chest compressions lead to questionable heart rhythms displayed on the monitor as someone shouts, "CHARGE!" Paddles are placed on the patient's chest as everyone scatters in response to "CLEAR!" Soon a full-court press of medication is released from the crash cart to whip the heart into further submission.

I am certain that most people never fully appreciate the level of attachment maintained to loved ones, places or keepsakes until they are swept away at the end of life. Items can be replaced and memories sustained, but the loss of life is never replaced. In reality, life is not the same after losing those who sustain our lives. Patients are reluctant to be counted out and wish to remain among the living. As social beings, serious physical impairment creates the mental imperative to not separate from the herd. One of the great fears in dying is feeling torn from others.

The intimacy that two people enjoy when finishing the other's sentences becomes stifled when one is dying. Hesitation occurs in completing any sentence about dying, honoring death wishes, or voicing supportive words that suggest it is okay to die. Serious illness forces us to deal with our own mortality and vulnerability, triggering an awkward connection between loved one and patient. With respect to the dying, we find it difficult to say, "It's all right for you to pass" without conveying the impression that patients are worthless or useless. We build our life on the prospect of being useful; finding value in being useless is almost impossible.

People's worst fears often revolve around becoming lonely or betrayed. Those who fear betrayal tend to remain single, while those who fear loneliness often believe Alfred Lord Tennyson's quote, "It is better to have loved and lost than never to have loved at all." People enter into a relationship with the hope of living happily ever after. However, forces in nature work against that bliss, challenging faithfulness. Imperative to relationships is developing the ability to maintain a firm grip while not holding on too tightly. The fear of letting go within the context and language of love provides insights and rules of engagement. Reconciling the prospect of death within the capacity to love will challenge any relationship.

In his book *The 5 Love Languages,* Gary Chapman addresses the confusion that occurs in relationships when couples attempt to communicate romantic love in different languages. His premise is that relationships require language consistent with words and actions that fill each other's *love tank.* The *love tank* is supplied by five pipelines of flattery or affection including Words of Affirmation, Quality Time, Receiving Gifts, Acts of Service and Physical Touch.[9] Knowing which language of love makes the world go round translates into fear once our world stops and separation anxiety takes hold.

For example, a friend of mine knows she is loved whenever someone does an act of service for her, such as cleaning the house, preparing a meal, mowing the lawn or folding laundry. While she considers cooking something special for her husband an act of love, he is forlorn in the bedroom—with a different act of love on his mind. Actions that wish to demonstrate love require we know our audience. When another friend was dying of a debilitating neurological disease, I arranged for daily massages to be provided by a therapist. Sending flowers may have been nice, but massages better replenished his *love tank.*

Whatever language fills the *love tank* and fuels lives easily translates into the language of fear when the tank springs a leak. When hearing words of disease, demise or death, it becomes difficult to find words that appease. Words may not be enough when situations become unbelievable and unspeakable. As quality time becomes cut short, there is more alone time. We can easily bide time rather than appreciate the remaining time. With time being of the essence and essential to filling the *love tank,* hearing "Time's up" damages the psyche.

When receiving gifts directly influences how much we are loved, the prospect of no more gifts becomes devastating. Acts of service bestow a figurative badge of honor on a purposeful life. Stewards of love expect to receive a reasonable return on any investment of service: "If I scratch your back, you scratch mine." When we are no longer able to care for others or ourselves, being of service becomes less than rewarding, purposeless and life ending. When nothing says, "I love you" like making love or receiving a hug, the restraining order issued by crippling disease often results in performance anxiety or alienation of affection.

Love of life rapidly becomes lost in fear as the love tank becomes filled with the alternative fuel of deprivation along with self-deprecation. This watered-down fuel, lacking positive words, time, gifts, services and physical attention does not mix well with efforts to energize and endear the spirit. With self-esteem in jeopardy, fear upsets and displaces quality of life with an insufferable way of life.

When there is dignity in certainty and no certainty in anxiety, there is no dignity in anxiety. I can attest to caring for a multitude of anxious patients, yet few of these maintain dignity. Anxiety feels like being trapped in a persistent state of impending doom. It greatly impedes listening, decision-making capacity and certainty. Amid the experience of separation anxiety there is an opportunity to *pause, center and shift,* separating and discerning the issues that contribute to the anxiety.

As written in Ecclesiastes 3:1—*For everything there is a season, and a time for every purpose under heaven.* Equating the SAD of Separation Anxiety Disorder to a Seasonal Affective Directive might imply limiting time spent on being anxious to one season. Anxiety better serves as an occasional spice to life used in moderation. However, I observe people thriving on it, much like caffeine. Anxiety in conjunction with fear creates a survival instinct. As the end of life draws near, fear intensifies and impairs judgment. This determines which extremes will be given to prolong life. Anxiety mixed with fear leads to irrational and foolish decisions, pain and suffering.

WISH 23:

Pro-Life Anger Management

If the goal of Advance Care Directives is to reduce pain and suffering, then pain management might include anger management. Anger consumes lives as it sucks the dignity from being reasonable. Anger management calls for a plan to deal with the emotional turmoil of fear, competition, and separation anxiety. A disabling condition easily triggers loss of control. The question becomes: What can be done to manage the stress, fear and anger working against dignity? I am convinced that Advance Care Directives cannot be successfully enacted until emotions are managed rationally.

Pre-planning end-of-life choices while appropriately managing anger is how we learn to deal with situations in stride. It is important to get in touch and own our anger, since it can trigger undue stress. I ascribe to the advice, "Don't get mad; get even." The best channel of revenge from the perspective of becoming even is to level the playing field before enacting long-range plans. Anger management eases the escalation of tension. While remembering to *pause, center and shift*, I create the wherewithal and game plan to ease suffering.

I experienced the power of "ease" while receiving energy work from a chiropractor. He put me through a series of strength tests and informed me that my rib cage was out of whack. The chiropractor stated that this misalignment was affecting my back and limiting neck mobility. I was instructed to lie prone on the examination table while he reweaved my energy and left the room. I patiently waited and waited and waited some more, anticipating a spine adjustment. When he returned to repeat the strength tests, my whacked-out chest had realigned simply through relaxation. His theory was that the body has an innate sense of healing and the ability to regain strength when allowing for "ease."

Similar to speeding on the freeway, we strive to get ahead in life and arrive at our final destination expeditiously. Most realize over time that we can reach the same destination with much less stress while taking it easy and creating more peace. The power to enact Advance Care Directives could arise from anger or solace. Which seems more heart-centered? Illness tends to be unexpected like being stabbed in the back. Believing mind, body and soul have been betrayed leads to an *Et-tu-Brute* moment of raw emotion. This can result in crimes of passion that sabotage actual kindheartedness toward illness afflicting the body.

The anguish of dying leaves us feeling forsaken, abandoned and ready to lash out. Through engaging the heart's attribute of compassion, we have an inordinate vessel from which to ease stress. Channeling anger through compassion results in a successful remedy to deal with stress.

Stress becomes hidden in coping mechanisms. Anger management is not necessary for people in denial of stress. In fact, many angry patients in the ED deny being stressed. While attempting to call attention to their stress, anger erupts in the command, "Thou shalt not call it stress!" Through bargaining, patients acquiesce to plea deals. They will admit to being stressed as long as it does not imply they are crazy. Stress wears patients down until they become depressed, drained emotionally and physically. Remorsefully, stress has gotten the best of them. Acceptance of stress as unmanageable allows patients to become more resourceful through compassion and ease.

Dignity becomes derailed when defaulting to instinctive coping mechanisms. Proceeding full steam ahead to sustain life creates opposition to death, uncertainty and additional stress. When utilizing anger as a management style, we essentially enact misalignment, mismanagement and manipulation. This is counterproductive to any desire for a peaceful outcome. Anger is the perceived red light that we repeatedly encounter at the end of life. Hitting every red light can prevent proceeding smoothly to the intended destination.

As in the rules of the road—or the enactment of Advance Care Directives—the expectation is not to hit every red light along the way. The perceived persecution escalates anger. Proceeding toward the end of life, do red lights present an impasse or opportunity? Do they provide a moment to *pause, center and shift*? Paused at these recurrent intersections, the opportunity allows for one to proceed through the light frantic, turn left to commit suicide or turn right to access the heart. Anger will find an escape route. Therefore, Advance Care Directives require escape valves. Having a plan in place to deal with "road rage" lessens the chance of driving recklessly.

Uncertainty escalates stress into panic attacks or desperate acts. Certainty is found in the heart in the form of compassion. Anger feels like having no choice, particularly when diagnosed with a terminal illness. The gift of compassion allows for choice. Compassion is in constant arbitration with the mind's notion of survival of the fittest, negotiating an acceptance of death. Compassion softens passion, allowing us to pull back from the brink of despair while choosing to ease out of life gracefully.

WISH 24:

Pro-Choice Evolution

Before signing into the Emergency Department, many people have hit a wall of bewilderment. Their medical condition is not improving or has become worse. ED visits are wake-up calls that provide an opportunity to *pause, center and shift*, allowing for certainty to be addressed. Enacting Advance Care Directives could include an injunction to ease up before hitting the wall. When life-threatening situations occur, we tend to set plans in motion that can differ greatly from what is appropriate or realistic. Actually, we might wish to lighten up and approach the situation with less intensity. In effect, how we react in emergency situations will either advance pain and suffering or ease it.

Countless times I have stood with patients and family members at the crossroads of life and death. They can no longer manage and wish for me to correct the futile situation. I assess the patient on the deathbed clinging to life and simply wonder why anyone would stop this patient from dying. Family members honestly believe more treatment is needed. However, additional treatment would be intrusive, obtuse and even potentially worse than the disease. It never feels right to inflict unimaginable pain on patients in order to make family members feel better.

Whatever comes naturally appears easy; becoming ill is naturally easy. The dis-ease that comes with illness is the undying belief that it is unnatural. Certainty is born from what comes naturally. Compassion affords being pro-choice regarding illness being natural. Having pain is inevitable, but suffering remains optional.

We bargain with ourselves and others, proclaiming, "We can do this the easy way or the hard way." Most people prefer the easy way. Unfortunately, dying becomes difficult when considered contrary to human life. Bargaining with death begins with an appreciation that dying is innately a part of living. What appears naturally instinctive circulates from the heart as *innate harmony*. Advance Care Directives arising from the heart incorporate the attribute of *innate harmony* into the process of dying. Pro-choice involves going with the flow or working against nature.

Before entering a department store, reasonable people have an idea of how much time and money they are willing to spend. Knowing how much an item should cost balanced against how much we are willing to spend above its cost is what dignity affords. Exiting the department store with our heads held high rather than in defeat is how most of us wish to exit life— consciously aware that we stuck with our intention and plan. The certainty of being right evolves easily when events unfold in our favor. We find an item on sale, win the jackpot or recover from an illness quickly. When the stakes are high, risks are great and there is no guarantee of winning amid having a lot to lose. The certainty of right becomes a crapshoot.

To simplify the process and dignify the right of passage, we might apply critical thinking to both bargaining and batting. Keeping an eye on the "throes" at the end of life is like keeping our eye on the ball. We need to look for pitched balls within the strike zone, stepping back from those above and beyond the range of a dignified swing. The one-two pitch of risk combined with prudence affects being pro-choice with suffering or survival.

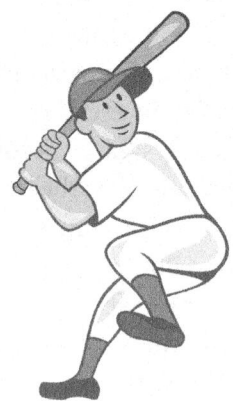

WISH 25:

Pro-Choice Survival Rule of Threes

If suddenly cast on the TV show *Survivor*, my Advance Care Directive Survival Guide would include and apply the survival rule of threes. Emphasized in the guide, priority and preparedness are necessary to survival awareness. This awareness provides for peace of mind and eases undue suffering through increments of three:

- 3 minutes without air (in lieu of suffering, I opt for suffocation)
- 3 hours without shelter (in lieu of suffering, I opt for exposure)
- 3 days without water (in lieu of suffering, I opt for dehydration)
- 3 weeks without food (in lieu of suffering, I opt for starvation)
- 3 months without hope (in lieu of suffering, I opt for hopelessness)

The harsh concepts of suffocation, exposure, dehydration, starvation and hopelessness may seem like cruel and unusual punishment for the living. For those dying, the jury still is out as to whether these allow for mercy. Which seems more dignified: Prolonged suffering or death by suffocation, exposure, dehydration, starvation or hopelessness? Actually, all of these are natural causes of death. They are also reversible, but will prolong life and suffering. Attempting to correct these reversible conditions could run counter to my intention and certainty of being right to die of natural causes.

I frequently question, "What are we treating here?" I believe unnecessary treatment prevents natural causes from allowing patients to pass. The enactment of my Advance Care Directive begins with the conscious effort to improve my medical situation. However, when illness prevails, I will bargain with healthcare providers to allow me to endure suffocation, exposure, dehydration, starvation, and hopelessness through being sedated and unconscious. I give priority to patients who are suffering, especially when they are suffocating. However, I might recommend sedation rather than specific medications that would reverse the respiratory distress associated with dying and prolong their suffering.

Permission is granted to enact Advance Care Directives when a terminal illness or persistent vegetative state is diagnosed. With the survival rule of threes as my rule of thumb, I advance my plan of action through three attempts or increments of time. I intend to use my rule of thumb at each benchmark to renegotiate the strategy, depending upon success or failure in conjunction with quality of life. If unable to live semi-independently, I wish to defer advance medical care. A bargain results in deal or no deal—*give me liberty or give me death*. Death is to be granted mercifully by allowing natural causes to enact their course.

During cardiac arrest there is an algorithm of threes that supports being for or against survival:

- 3 immediate shocks to the heart
- 3-minute intervals of epinephrine administered three times
- 30 minutes of CPR without regaining a pulse negates survival

Most people are averse to the idea of being electrocuted. If it becomes necessary to jumpstart my heart with an electric jolt, I prefer to pass. Similarly, I would rather not have artificial intravenous adrenaline (epinephrine) flog my heart. When it is time to die, let my heart rest. Thirty minutes of CPR, or what I perceive as "Chaotic Purposeless Righteousness," is unnecessary when I prefer to die. We spend much of our lives with the wish to die suddenly, but CPR is initiated in most cardiac arrests. The tendency is to fight against the heart's inclination to stop beating and bargain for more time.

In applying the algorithm of the survival rule of threes, I hear, "Three strikes; you're out." The link to America's favorite pastime determines when I am past time. Throughout life, every day we figuratively step in the batter's box. Dignity is on the line at that moment, with all eyes on the batter. When the pitch is thrown, we plant our feet—chin up, knees bent—and keep our eyes on the ball. We swing with all our strength. The batter's hope is to connect with the ball and send it flying. When faced with a terminal illness, any hit could get us to first base on the way to remission or recovery. When striking out, we leave the batter's box willingly. Being a good sport advances the certainty of being right.

To incessantly ask for more pitches would be considered unsportsmanlike and undignified. Having batters remain in the box until they get a hit would be badgering and abusive. Advance Care Directives might include the statement that if remission is not achieved following three separate treatments, it is not meant to be. If it takes three weeks to break a habit and three jolts to restart the heart, three attempts or three increments of anything give us ample opportunity to *pause, center and shift*. When Advance Care Directives become activated with the diagnosis of a terminal illness or a persistent vegetative state, what type of increment or rule of three is reasonable before the right to die is definitively granted with mercy, certainty and dignity?

Not wishing to suffer for the long haul reminds us that God only permitted Christ to fall three times in His passion and death. With respect to cardiac disease, perhaps we draw the line at three cardiac resuscitations, three heart attacks, three cardiac procedures during a lifetime or three ED visits for chest pain within a year. With repeated respiratory distress, is a ventilator required three times over the course of a year or perhaps indefinitely for three months or three years? How long is remaining in a coma acceptable? Three days may be too soon to pull the plug. However, after three weeks, three months, three years or three decades, do we concede the possible miraculous awakening for the chance to pass with dignity?

The concept of having three strikes is not enough for some, but could offer peace of mind to others. Similarly, when three needle sticks fail to access a vein we prefer another nurse or course of direction. With any chronic illness comes the fear and frustration of relinquishing control. We cannot predict how long pain and suffering will continue. Many of us become caught up in the acceleration and exhilaration of fear, perhaps proceeding three miles beyond the intended exit. The floorboard of Advance Care Directives includes both accelerator and brake pedals.

Remaining at ease while driving requires vigilance and dexterity; we can hit the brakes to helplessness and the accelerator to cleverness.

I began to practice what I preach after sustaining a shoulder injury while snowboarding. The shoulder was not dislocated or broken, but suffered a significant blow. I questioned whether I should have an MRI, see an orthopedic physician or simply let it heal on its own. I wondered what an adequate period of healing might be: three days, three weeks, three months or longer? Three days would be an unrealistic timeframe for adequate recovery. I did not want to enact treatment that might potentially sabotage the body's natural ability to heal. Certainty allowed me to give my shoulder several three-month periods of strengthening exercises before receiving a steroid injection.

When a cancerous lesion was noted on my father's bladder during an abdominal CT scan, I was reluctant to make mention of it and even less interested in having it treated. I supported his desire to be viewed as healthy despite the physical debilitation of peripheral neuropathy. My certainty was outvoted by other family members certain that the presumed cancer needed to be addressed. A biopsy determined the lesion was malignant—and those family members insisted on treatment. He was scheduled for six three-week rounds of BCG immunotherapy treatment. I outlined a protocol in conjunction with the survival rule of threes—he was to receive three weeks of treatment and have his tolerance to chemotherapy assessed. After two of the three-week rounds of therapy he was extremely weak and treatment ceased. Of note, four years later he has sustained no ill effects from not continuing treatment.

Cancer treatment has advanced tremendously in recent years and oncologists offer a wide array of aggressive treatment options. The bread and butter of an oncologist's practice are the pursuit of aggressive treatment and preserving life. This satisfies patients who buy into the notion that physicians are to never give up, regardless of the circumstances. In the fight to save lives and guard salvation, we are tempted not to stop any treatment. By declining further treatment, patients often feel condemned by going against the recommendation of physicians who appears to be Godlike. When do patients receive permission to stop treatment?

The illusion of what an oncologist can and cannot do to sustain life leads many patients to the waiting room of the Emergency Department, weighing the prospect of survival against the next best treatment in the queue. Part of my responsibility as an EM physician requires discerning whether survival is unlikely or unrealistic. Ineffective results after three months' time aids my certainty and might lessen a patient's hope for survival.

In cancer treatment, the three possible interventions presented to patients include surgery, radiation or chemotherapy. At the outset of treatment, doctors follow protocols regarding doses, timeframes and time intervals that gauge results with regard to reevaluation and redirection of treatment. Once again, my thinking is not along the lines of unlimited treatment, but simply the survival rule of threes that intends to ultimately limit hope.

WISH 26:

Pro-Choice in the Context of Hope

While exercising our bargaining rights, hope releases endorphins. Hope runs eternal as we embark on the marathon to save life. Hope could be visualized by the Energizer Bunny weaving a trail across a casino floor beating its drum, intent on beating the odds. This escape from reality is the gamble fueled by passion and faith. Whereas faith emerges from thoughts and beliefs, hope pulsates from the heart that is impervious to shame. The heart knows no bounds, generating hope as though there is a surplus of options and tomorrows.

Hope flows freely and unconditionally from the heart, ranging from the extremes of being free of illness to accepting death. Lessening the passion of hope with more *innate harmony* from the heart leads to serenity. The heart receives input from both right and left sides of the brain; creative energy and scientific thinking co-exist respectively within the psyche. The right mindset of wishful thinking adds to suffering when expectation is steeped in hope. The left mindset sends impulses that can enact a change of heart and perhaps detonate hope. By turning the spigot of hope clockwise, suffering can be eased.

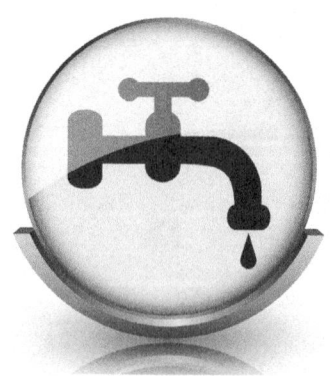

When patients lie dormant in the intensive care unit, there is rarely respect given to the disease process or the person fit to be tied to technology. In every physician's mind are the words of slain activist and San Francisco Supervisor Harvey Milk, "You gotta give 'em hope." Patients and their families expect to receive hope from physicians. Physicians, who can be faulted for providing too much hope or giving too much hype. Expectations are rarely clarified or dignified when the reality of a cure is outside the realm of possibility. Believing I can turn back the hands of time rarely honors the disease process or dignity itself. I don't expect my father's health to significantly improve—yet I encourage him to enjoy what he can still do without imposing false beliefs.

Hope is the physician's best marketing tool for enacting treatment, second only to instilling guilt. A physician seemingly eases patients' end-of-life concerns by billing them through PayPal account of hope. Any promise disallows skepticism or pessimism. Left-brain skepticism will be countered by an equal and opposing "Hail Mary pass" or miracle conjured up by the right brain. Blind faith fosters heroic measures that lead to doing everything and anything possible to survive. According to the survival rule of threes, hope lasts for three months. I concur that in the absence of hope after three months, hanging on seems unreasonable. Hope runs eternal, especially in the face of patients becoming unconscious. If conscious, most people would never wish to have their lives prolonged in a coma or persistent vegetative state beyond a three-month period.

Hope needs to remain detached from expectation and outcome. I particularly emphasize this when individuals undertake weight-loss programs. People begin these programs with the intention of losing weight rather than approach their goals from a health-conscious, heart-centered perspective. In reality, diets are not health-conscious patterns of eating. What is good for the heart is also good for mind and body. Weight adjusts as cardiovascular exercise is implemented and metabolism reinvigorated. I use the same "law of detachment," or hope without expectation, in regard to my calf workouts. I never expect my calves to get bigger, but keep hope in my exercise program that includes calf raises to strengthen my Achilles heel.

Making the best of a bad situation is not achieved through hope, but rather through enlightenment. The wisdom of enlightenment eases the suffering of hopelessness through detachment. A hopeless illness is potentially a gift taken to heart. The heart's *innate harmony* ultimately affirms the rite of passage to dying with dignity. We gain from having an illness, such as a stronger immune system or greater resolve. We rarely bargain to be afflicted with a disease, but we have the capacity to become better people as an illness progresses. True to my experience, some of the nicest people I meet are the sickest patients.

Tears shed from an overflow of emotions stream from both sorrow and gratitude. When we *pause, center and shift* from tears of grief to gratitude, we awaken to the idea that gratitude immediately shifts the focus from sadness to appreciation. Tears from sorrow enlist a cry for help, more treatment and more attention. Offering up suffering for the greater good releases the need for more attention and increases the certainty of being right with what life has given. The more suffering becomes optional, the less overall suffering is endured. We leave the world a better place through letting go of suffering and focusing more on thanksgiving.

Few of us wish to believe life is all for naught. Sadly, many people see nothingness at the end of life. We may see our lives as a harvest remembered for a season and then forgotten. Advance Care Directives remind us of the bargain to reap what we sow. How the seed of dignity is planted in our directives determines how we reap dignity at the end of life. The less certainty contained in our directives, the less dignity becomes enacted. The spiritual harvest from living comes from being thankful for life. When we ease up and enact our directives from a place of thanksgiving, we are less likely to be led into temptation. The greatest temptation at the end of life is to perceive death as evil, hoping and praying for deliverance from it.

We are tempted to sell our souls to a healthcare system intent on sustaining life at any cost while losing dignity. From the certainty of being right, I prefer to barter with a healthcare system that supports my dignity. The devil in the healthcare system sells treatments that encourage wishful thinking. Waiting for a miracle may prolong suffering and bargain away dignity. There is more to fear than meets the eye when tempting fate, yet few of us see the temptation behind the fear that enhances pain and suffering.

The doors to the Emergency Department automatically slide open and invite us to experience fewer options and more of what the healthcare system offers. Established core measures, assigned duties, questions of negligence and the need for compliance create conflicts between providing the right measures for the wrong reasons. Temptation is the desire to have or do something that you know should be resisted. Requesting pain medication under the guise of embellished pain often compromises personal responsibility, principle and proper conduct. The physician's written prescription can become a permission slip to ignore the risk of narcotic dependency and its consequences. While attempting to avoid harmful predicaments, we often unconsciously attract what we fear. Mark Twain asserts, "There are several good protections against temptation, but the surest is cowardice."

Facing serious illness puts us to the test. The healthcare system will tempt us with secondary gains including increased attention, disability benefits and the release from personal responsibilities. There is the temptation to use illness to manipulate others and situations. Through fear that leads to temptation, we are apt to reach for another treatment or more second opinions. We may become artful at self-medicating, while unconsciously actuating more fear of dependency and enrolling others in enabling secondary gains. This self-fulfilling attraction to suffering can distract patients from both healing and certainty.

The temptation to hold on to life determines our actions as the end draws near. Fear leads to irrational behavior, allowing for foolish decisions. I was considering refinancing my home mortgage with an offer that appeared too good to be true. The chance of realizing a principle reduction to my mortgage was similar to the chance of my actually winning the Publishers Clearing House sweepstakes. The principle reduction program was much more about seduction than reduction. In wanting a quick fix, I began to believe it was true.

The dirty little secret about entering a rehabilitation center is that it often leads to an indefinite stay in an extended-care facility. Most people continue to swear they are never going to end up in one of these facilities as they are being wheeled through its doors. The clever patient negotiates the terms of stay at admission. If I were to reside there longer than three months, my recovery plan would be redirected to my end-of-life plan. This plan includes avoiding any forced preventive measures, medications, or provisions that might prolong my life. My Advance Care Directive is not to be enacted indefinitely. It contains benchmarks as guidelines. When Advance Care Directives only propose continuing to live, I observe patients bargaining for more time or a better outcome. If these undying initiatives were not addressed when the patient was in good health, they lose bargaining power while confined in an extended-care facility.

I choose to *pause, center and shift* my decision-making in the present moment to anticipate future dilemmas. I realize a DNR today would not be upheld due to my age and not having a terminal illness. In the present moment I could defer on receiving a flu shot, but my livelihood demands it. I continue to debate the cost benefit of having an age-appropriate colonoscopy in relation to my dignity. My certainty of being right tells me I do not have colon cancer. Enacting my survival rule of threes, I will reconsider the merits of this procedure in another three years.

The concept of bargaining creates an awareness of the middle ground between life and death. We hold onto our wishes, but need to be flexible as circumstances change. We consider letting go, but not too soon. Certainty is best experienced while remaining centered. Seeking to reclaim our center through each step of the dying process permits us to *live and let die.* My Advance Care Directive emphasizes my desire to maintain moderation and encourages caregivers to provide less temptation and more moderation when treating chronic illness or injury.

We cannot plan for car accidents, heart attacks and strokes, but we can acknowledge the possibility of an unexpected crisis and have a plan to address it. How would we respond to a poor prognosis? A doctor solicits direction from the patient or family members as to how they wish to proceed. People may long for certainty when the end of life is near, but few people ever wish to hear life-saving measures are futile. I welcome the concept of futility as my greatest bargaining strategy to dying with dignity. A physician's certainty of imminent demise provides the certainty of being right with permission to stop unnecessary treatments.

When the chips are down and healthcare providers are called upon to save a life or spare dignity, do we remember with certainty that dignity is of the utmost importance? When saving my life comes down to a question rather than a given, I am mindful of the warning: "This has been a test of the Emergency Broadcast System . . . in an actual emergency, you will be instructed to tune to a station in your area for updated news and official information." When the news is challenging, what do we tune into and what official information is required? In an emergency, we can interrupt this life-saving announcement by hitting the pause button, easing into the center and shifting toward a cause for dignity.

I am certain about my own course. I do not wish to prolong suffering in a futile attempt to save my life. In its enactment, my Advance Care Directive completely waives my right to be saved when unable to speak for myself. Some choose to fight until the end; I wish to be treated with the certainty that dignity will pave my path to the end. I look to my own center, not one imposed by others. I will not bargain for perpetuity, but to attain grace under fire, forbearance without perseverance, liberty in lieu of longevity, and to forsake everything in the quest for dignity.

The bargain at the end of life weighs the time remaining. Terminal illness presents the challenge to view and reprioritize life to achieve a sense of completion. Caregivers need to know the focus is no longer on saving my life, but on my dying gracefully. I cared for a patient with lung cancer who was having a rough time. I suggested he have "the talk" with his family and let them know he was ready to die. Two weeks later he was readmitted to the ED and informed me that his family was not ready to let him go. They told him to forget about dying. I wondered what might have been miscommunicated or misconstrued in his wishes.

People are normally uncomfortable talking about dying. The center of certainty often becomes disregarded an actions are taken that usurp patients' comfort. Any enactment of Advance Care Directives needs to anticipate these hardships. The bargain I make is to endure the hardship just long enough to realize the direction I am headed toward. Bargaining is over when the point of no return is crossed; the only option I want left on the table is peace of mind. Given this benchmark, I only need to be conscious long enough to make dying mindful, meaningful and certain.

WISH 27:

Pro-End-of-Life Revelation

What goes up must come down. The higher the expectation, the harder it is to accept disappointment. The enactment of Advance Care Directives requires courage and receptivity to revelation. We know the body is engineered to eventually fail, but it is depressing to realize one has become old, tired and ill. The mind perceives aging as having less strength, as though growing older and weaker are shameful. The body is apt to give out while the mind remains adamant about not giving up. Many elderly succumb to this predicament through depression. This sinking feeling leads to a dark place that envisions life slipping away while circling the drain.

Fighting back feels like treading water. This process, inherent to dying, will drain us emotionally and physically. It is impossible to hold on indefinitely during this sink-or-swim dilemma. The best option for dealing with depression is composing our thoughts with the certainty of being right. Depression can be a means to an end, perhaps shifting the focus of enacting Advance Care Directives to ending life. This shift can override depression through stewardship. Running a rototiller over the perceived wrongs in life prepares the soil for planting seeds. The revelation of spring awakening will sprout from depression.

While contemplating an end-of-life plan, there is a strong temptation to slip into depression. Whether it causes illness or is the result of it, depression holds us back from living life to the fullest. When we are dying, depression naturally becomes a deeper distraction through the need to withdraw inward. Depression triggers giving up the will to live. We lose sight of what really matters, letting go of loved ones and activities enjoyed. My Advance Care Directive has a somewhat Buddhist philosophy that invites me to "love without attachment," not allowing the anchor of depression to drag me further into deep waters.

As life expectancy diminishes, we tend to expect to live exactly the number of years predicted, as if this were a lifetime guarantee. Why not focus on living those remaining years with the highest quality of life possible? We re-read the lifetime contract and realize it comes with many disclaimers associated with accidental occurrences. The truth is that we do not necessarily have precise expiration dates. We are not entitled to four-score years and ten, or whatever life expectancy our parents experienced. This false claim of entitlement built into the concept of life expectancy leaves us looking for someone to blame when our time is cut short. By negating responsibility for our lives and believing illness excuses us from being responsible, we default to becoming victims of illness. A helpless attitude will lead to further depression.

To be labeled with depression gives the impression that our decision-making capacity has been compromised. Decisions made under the duress of depression become suspect. Therefore, others will assume responsibility for our lives. The sabotaging effects of depression typically invalidate impromptu personal wishes that were not provided for in Advance Care Directives. Ideally, Advance Care Directives have a natural evolution to their enactment that culminates in a pro-end- of-life revelation. Depression aids this revelation and is a natural catalyst to withdrawing from life. Recognizing depression as being a necessary evolution to the end of life advances the certainty of being right when becoming depressed.

The uncertainty inherent to depression permits people to be less responsible. However, the concept of dignity combats irresponsibility by opening the door to possibilities. Although I do not personally advocate for physician-assisted suicide, I do appreciate it as means for people to be responsible for their deaths. Choice affords empowerment while no choice leads to depression. Wishing to not become depressed is useless. Wishing to move life beyond the stagnation felt with depression emboldens people.

At the intersection of depression and dignity, the certainty of a right-of-way merges with the rite of passage to death. It is always fascinating to observe those at the crossroads who assert their right-of-way, wave others ahead or seem to be sleeping at the wheel. The rules of the road determine the proper time to proceed through the intersection. People who choose not to claim their right-of-way due to diminished self-importance and lack of certainty frustrate me. At the intersection of life and death, having the right-of-way is ideally a prospective rather than a retrospective decree of "I should have gone." I generally perceive an Advance Care Directive as a one-way tunnel hell-bent on survival, perhaps with tunnel vision. Having dignity allows me to perceive the light the end of the tunnel, but depression will feel like hitting a dead end.

In a persistent depressive state we lose our sense of dignity and direction. Depression, like a creative detour off the main road, may add a scenic perspective to life and an opportunity to be inspired. We could actually use this opportunity to *pause, center and shift* the perception of negativity to creativity. Cautious optimism is the safest course. Otherwise, we risk mood swings between positive and negative forces that contribute to uncertainty when hopes and dreams are dashed. Survival is built on a foundation of guarded, realistic optimism.

I caution cancer survivors to remain vigilant and prudent once they achieve remission or are deemed cancer free, since cancer propagates itself. Over-exuberance can serve as a defense to mask fear, depression or other negative energy. My friend, Gwen, placed her hopes solely on her husband's survival of multiple myeloma. Once he attained remission, he oddly slumped further into depression. The revelation of no longer being invincible—along with the looming threat of cancer on the horizon—hung like a dark cloud over his head.

Life's journey is comprised of statistics, benchmarks and algorithms set up like brackets in a basketball tournament. Individuals, like teams, are seeded as to who is most likely to succeed. The tournament of life begins with high hopes or poor prospects due to genetic engineering, level of conditioning and luck. Our preamble determines whether our own personal tournament enacts a single elimination, double elimination or the unlimited chances to advance in the brackets. Envisioning dignity as "double or nothing" allows me to set up my tournament with a double elimination. The first defeat will occur with diagnosis of a life-threatening disease and the second loss in the consolation bracket will arise with recurrence of the life-threatening disease. Treatment is optional at this point since I will give consideration to palliative care.

Following the second loss, I will have one last shot for a "new lease on life" before *game over*. Once diagnosed with a terminal illness, I can no longer claim my health status as being undefeated. Once relegated to the consolation bracket, *game on!*

TOURNAMENT OF LIFE

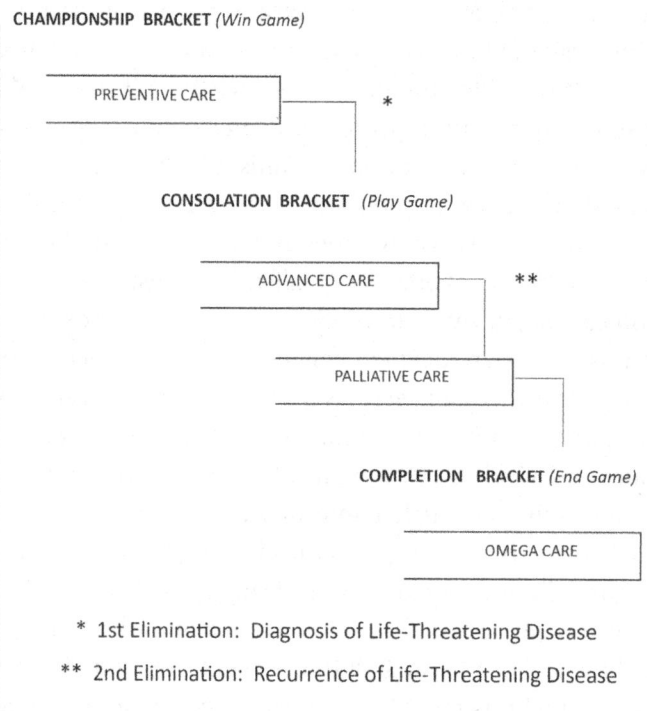

CHAMPIONSHIP BRACKET *(Win Game)*

PREVENTIVE CARE

*

CONSOLATION BRACKET *(Play Game)*

ADVANCED CARE

**

PALLIATIVE CARE

COMPLETION BRACKET *(End Game)*

OMEGA CARE

* 1st Elimination: Diagnosis of Life-Threatening Disease

** 2nd Elimination: Recurrence of Life-Threatening Disease

Gwen's husband prided himself on having excellent health until multiple myeloma positioned him into the consolation bracket. Naturally, we become depressed momentarily when forced into the consolation bracket. Experiencing anything less than winning while remaining undefeated has inherent upsets. However, the consolation bracket has its own merits of humility with decidedly less focus on winning. *It's not whether you win or lose, it's how you play the game.* The championship bracket focuses on winning; the consolation bracket focuses on playing the game and emphasizes quality of life. A wonderful reprise to actually enjoying life is no longer feeling compelled to win.

WISH 28:

Pro-End-of-Life Survival Instinct Unplugged

Whether having survived cancer or a heart attack, we typically return to the playing field with the eye of a tiger focused on survival. We are challenged by fear and soothed in consolation. The first wave of fear in a life-threatening situation triggers anger. The second wave of fear hides in depression. Bob Lonsberry, author of *A Various Language* states, "Fear is a quicksand that slows and grips and strangles [similar to depression], leaving its victims unable to act."[10] Do we expect to be become consumed and buried by depression before life ends? In my Advance Care Directive, I appreciate depression as consolation over fear. I wish to die in this contentment rather than engulfed by the depression that seemingly enacts a sad ending.

Depression is not always obvious. People would rather not admit to being depressed, given its societal stigma. Many suffer in silence, while others remedy the situation with anti-depressants. When people around us experience depression, the inclination is to cheer them up rather than allow them to remain depressed. Optimism and sweeteners provide a contrasting flavor to the perceived bitterness associated with dying. There is a strong tendency for terminal illness to be sugarcoated in the current delivery of healthcare. Sugarcoating the harsh reality of death is detrimental to dignity and needs to be unplugged. Many of us have a sweet tooth and will suffer the consequence of having a blood sugar crash.

Abstaining from sugar tends to increase craving sugar. Similarly, being deprived or denied a future tends to incur craving a longer life. When depression leads to withdrawal, we need to enact Advance Care Directives that unplug dependency from depression. Depression leads to detachment, while dependency sustains attachment. Depressed patients frequently imbibe alcohol and/or narcotics. Therefore, dependency may lead to withdrawing from life cold turkey. During this separation process, people experience agitation, tears, sweating, nausea, muscle aches and fatigue—along with palpitations and sleep disturbances. These withdrawal symptoms only complicate and worsen the depression associated with dying.

Advance Care Directives strive for fulfillment; depression normally contributes to feeling unfulfilled. Depression can cause a free fall into dependency, hopelessness and helplessness. Sadness often results from falling short of expectation, or illness taking precedence over life. Depression may also lead to withdrawal from normal activities or vengeful behavior like self-mutilation or substance abuse. Dis-ease associated with chronic pain may also lead to substance abuse. Studies have shown that long-term (more than three months) reliance on pain medication often leaves patients permanently dependent on narcotics that have depressive side effects.

Dependency only serves to compound the experience of depression. Placing dignity aside, we may have other pressing issues that need to be addressed when dependent on relationships, substances, appearances or worthiness. These dependencies often compensate for inadequacies that compel us to attempt to raise self-image or get high. The fall from grace and loss of dignity occur when depression goes unrecognized beneath dependency. Dependency prompts an attachment to life while potentially leaving us powerless over death.

The enactment of Advance Care Directives begins with survival of the fittest (anger), progresses by the survival rule of threes (bargaining) and concludes by unplugging the survival instinct (depression). The transformation of depression from passively giving up to actively pulling the plug works to our advantage. During the end-of-life free fall, depression can be equivalent to pulling the ripcord and releasing the parachute to soften the landing. The paradox is that depression is a natural catalyst to letting go, which is a necessary evolution in enacting Advance Care Directives. The goal of my Advance Care Directive is to attain peace, not plummet solely into depression and experience life smashed to smithereens.

The enactment of Advance Care Directives will turn up the heat, similar to when instructors raise the heat in a hot yoga class. This is where I meet my Waterloo in a puddle of dripping sweat. Instructors often say that it is all right to give up and lie down on your mat. This encourages the unspeakable—that death is acceptable. However, what I hear is, "I dare you to let the class see how you give up when the heat is on." Rebelling against this perceived challenge, I attempt to remain upright while becoming denatured, drained of all my faculties and energies. When muscles break down or become denatured and neurons become like Jell-O, I actually care less. By ignoring the instructor's directions, my yoga practice becomes careless and sloppy.

Ideally, in life—as in the practice of yoga—I am cautious about reaching the point of annihilation and potentially becoming depleted of my natural ability. Depression presents two options regarding mortification of the flesh—becoming careless or becoming carefree. When the first maddening insult of a fatal diagnosis combines with the second infuriating assault of failed treatment, why bother to care period? Being careless subjects me to a second wave of anger that is masked by passive-aggressive hostility. While overhearing a nurse badger a terminally ill patient to come to some decision about life support, I understood how I would react. Her aggression triggered my own thoughts of anger and careless retaliation. The patient chose to harm himself by seeking vengeance against the nurse through choosing life support.

In retrospect, this situation could have been approached differently by unplugging anger from aggression. Slipping into depression can trigger either overt anger or passive-aggressive behavior. While meltdowns are inevitable, both dispositions are careless. Fear of being mistreated or wronged generally leads to more harm being done. Transforming depression into a carefree state actually prompts being more careful with end-of-life decisions.

When Mamie was hospitalized for pneumonia and diagnosed with lung cancer, the discharge plan was for her to be admitted to an extended-care facility. The expectation was that she needed rest to prepare for upcoming chemotherapy. Staff at the long-term care facility promptly returned her to the Emergency Department, determining she was too lethargic to be managed there. Mamie was not lethargic; she was apathetic. She had been a proud, 70-year-old woman who looked 50 and was now withdrawn and depressed. I could see the glowing timbers of the fireball she had been. She was no longer engaged in life. Mamie did not speak to me, but I could tell she was listening intently as her daughter and I spoke freely. It was obvious she was not interested in chemotherapy. I simply offered her the option to unplug from what was expected of her in order to regain her spirited passion.

WISH 29:

Pro-End-of-Life Resolution

When choosing to do harm, we die hard, beaten down by our own depression. The self-harm that often occurs through the process of dying appears poisonous and might be represented by the skull and crossbones. Figuratively inscribed underneath the skull and crossbones is the captive phrase that is telltale of depression: *The beatings will continue until morale improves.* Naturally, morale fades as we wax, wane and denature at the end of life. Throughout the process of dying, the whip of opposition, hardship and suffering strikes repeatedly. According to sociologist and psychiatrist Alexander Leighton, MD, "Morale is the capacity of a group of people to pull together persistently and consistently in pursuit of a common purpose." However, the catch-22 that occurs from attempting to improve morale is that this encourages the beatings with resolutions to do more harm than good.

Raising morale seems to be right. Lifting spirits with pure intention, morale might collapse on the prospect of being moral. Nevertheless, the experience of depression projects an immoral image of being sullen and disconnected from ourselves. When receiving the diagnosis of terminal illness, we naturally confront mortality. Refusing to accept our own mortality can lead to depression. The more I accept my mortality, the less I need to improve my morale. "Enough already" is an appeal muttered by even semiconscious patients who understand that their physical and emotional needs can no longer be met by someone's misgivings. It never feels right to die until we are certain it is time to die. Then, the beatings can be deemed sufficient and come to an end.

What seems moral typically distinguishes right from wrong, but clarity given to dignity might help a patient assert that they are done with living rather than appearing down or depressed. Depression can end with the realization of being near the end of life, letting go of the fear surrounding mortality. After a phone conversation with my mother, listening to her complain about aches and pains, surgery or no surgery, pain medication or alternative medicine, wishing to change current living arrangements while not wishing to move, she sadly admitted, "I think I'm depressed." I could not help but think to myself, "Wait a minute, Mom, Before you slip too far into depression, please assert your dignity by telling me when you're done."

The second of my three wishes is for others to respect my dignity by allowing for free choice. I would like to extend the same respect to my mother whenever she becomes certain of being done. When I am dying, I want permission to be done. The dignity that emerges from this certainty allows me to announce—*I AM THAT I AM* (Exodus 3:14)—exactly where I am supposed to be while being depressed. When depressed, it feels like I am living a different existence than my norm and need to overcome it. If we believe death is to be overcome and that dying is wrong, how can we possibly envision the end of life with resolutions? Instead, we might believe that life events happen for a reason. Depression gives us another reason to *pause, center and shift* in considering the next stage of acceptance.

My father stumbled into the minefield of dependency after peripheral neuropathy left his arm and legs incapacitated through them being numb and weak. His uncertain gait compromised the surefootedness he had enjoyed in life and illustrated the fear of helplessness as when becoming more dependent upon caregivers. I thought my father would have been done with life when he reluctantly handed over the car keys and began sitting in the passenger seat. Instead, he resigned himself to being helpless and quietly depressed.

As family patriarch and Korean War veteran, my father had to decide whether to continue his battle for life with a signed DNR order. Living semi-independently with my mother in an assisted-living facility, he knew he was one step away from residing in a nursing home. Having always been adamantly opposed to dying in a nursing home, I thought he would readily accept and sign a DNR. Nevertheless, he was reluctant to sign it at the time. Irrationally, he is convinced that he can weather further challenges to his health without being wheeled into a nursing home.

I observe my father's decline in life, exacerbated by helplessness and depression. My mother, who only sees him sleeping all the time, missing the signs of depression. I see him sinking further in quicksand. He struggles every step of the way, still very much attached to life and stubbornly ignoring the signs of his increasing frailty. Previously, he was unable to bathe himself and would not ask for help. I tactfully reminded him that neglecting personal hygiene reflects poorly on his caregivers, who might be considered negligent. This lack of care could be reported as elder abuse. He acquiesced to being bathed by an aide and accepted my suggestion of considering these spa days.

Relying too heavily on others is characteristic of a dependent personality disorder (DPD). DPD increases the likelihood of abuse or dependence on alcohol or drugs. My father's situation illustrates the emotional turmoil between dependency and detachment. Being overly dependent, bordering on addiction, demeans personal coping skill and overall freedom. With the harsh reality that *it is what it is,* there is rarely a resolution to the duo of dependency and depression. To help others cope requires becoming complicit with their dependency. Unfortunately, this dependency stifles the certainty of being right.

We often surround ourselves with layers of emotional insulation in an attempt to create a protective wall against harm, annihilation and death. This structural support system is often fear-based, family-friendly, physician-directed and faith-inspired. Sinking in this quicksand of devastation, separation anxiety and desperation, it may be too late to be saved by others. People are apt to ignore the Hippocratic Oath to do no harm. Some people insist on action—anything to sustain life. I observe dependency impeding critical thinking and patient responsibility. Friends and family encourage patients to deny the prospect of dying through creating more dependency on caregivers.

Taking personal action with resolutions allows individuals to move beyond depression. Applying the same steps a person takes in following a twelve-step program sidesteps depression. The first step in the program is to admit we are powerless and life has become unmanageable. We might rise above depression by remembering the second step, which is to believe that a power greater than ourselves could restore us to sanity. Alcoholics Anonymous members famously proclaim, "Keep coming back. It works if you work it!" What I continually come back to is that a higher power has the ability to restore me to sanity, creating the prospect for dignity.

Depression and alcoholism are both rooted in powerlessness. Becoming helpless increases dependency on other persons, interventions, affirmations, and substances. People begin to question their ability to function without any of these support mechanisms. I realize personal power through maintaining quality of life which I perceive as deteriorating rapidly when I can no longer care for myself. Personal security gained from having freedom and choice provides a sense of control, power and resolutions to live carefree.

When diagnosed with serious illness or affliction, it is all too easy to lose this carefree attitude, stumbling into depression. A crucial misstep occurs through choosing not to manage ailments, addictions and afflictions. Similar to the progression of addiction, tolerance for depression increases. Friends and family seek another form of tolerance in dealing with their loved ones' afflictions. They may need to also admit powerlessness and unmanageability. When caring for a depressed person, I think to myself and sometimes suggest, "You are better than this." Dependency depletes certainty and the ability to maintain dignity. The path to dignity cannot be paved through dependency, helplessness and stubbornness.

I observe patients being completely inert at the end of life and unaffected by the swarm of activity around them. A swig of depression is one coping mechanism that clouds dependency issues. The new normal of terminal illness affords the choice of being flexible or stubborn.

When slipping further from independence, would Advance Care Directives have us make positive or negative resolutions? Dignity resides in the middle ground. Therefore, directives need to be aligned in the middle of being for or against end-of-life resolutions. Being inert typically suggests lifelessness, but I appreciate inert patients as being indifferent. Through indifference, patients might be grounded in a carefree zone of neutrality, contentment, certainty and perhaps sobriety.

While experiencing depression, life's transmission shifts from drive into neutral. The head naturally bows to the heart while shifting gears. Within the fog of depression the heart contains a pilot light with intrinsic inertia. If fueled properly, the heart ignites the premise that love heals all. "Love heals all" is validated when we recover. When not able to recover, depression ensues. The heart could recirculate the premise that love heals all to the transformative notion that love instills reconciliation. Reconciliation is appreciated through the heart's attribute of *healing presence*. This arbitrates the split between the mind-body connection that occurs when the body is weak but the mind remains strong.

Our minds become frustrated when our bodies ache, stagnate and can no longer perform to expectations. Conversely, our bodies deteriorate when lacking energy to properly take care of physical needs. The mind and the body are in conflict over living happily ever after or forever. Objectively, people in this dilemma admit themselves to the Emergency Department and plead for attention. In the ED, I may offer a moment of undivided attention to the situation at hand, but patients have to decide and resolve their management of illness and depression based on their own coping mechanisms.

People often recognize the mind-body connection being at odds within individuals who do not wish to die. The heart restores the mind-body connection by creatively combating helplessness. Mind and body need to join forces with the prospect of dying with dignity. When existing on divergent paths, the mind and body can be united through the heart, incorporating its *healing presence*. This requires the reverse psychology of proclaiming the weakest link as the greatest asset within the mind-body connection. This reminds me of the phrase, *The stone the builders rejected has become the cornerstone* (Psalm 118:22).

Depression feels like being stuck between a rock and a hard place. The rock of terminal illness weighs heavily upon us in the hard place of not wishing to let go of life. Therefore, we hit rock bottom. This predicament presents the opportunity to enact an end-of-life plan with a lasting legacy. Depression can leave us destitute; dignity calls us to contribute. The most profound way people give of themselves is through organ donation. Depression happens; how we deal with it is what matters most.

Depression leads to somber daydreams. As written in the Bible, what occurred to the Virgin Mary in a dream state was the Annunciation by the Angel Gabriel. I presume the same *annunciation* occurs within the dream state of terminal illness. Once the presumed *annunciation* occurs—upon receiving a poor prognosis in conjunction with terminal illness—do we become a servant like the Holy Mother of God? *Behold, I am the hand-maid of the Lord. May it be done to me according to your word* (Luke 1:38), becomes the voice of humility, dignity and resolution.

I see people flock to the Emergency Department for end-of-life care and wonder whether they received the memo from the Angel Gabriel. Wake Up People! We will not grasp the legitimacy of dying until we hear it from inside, perhaps through an end-of-life revelation while in a dream state. A peaceful death resolves to welcome the news with acceptance. Ultimately listening to the whispers of the lullaby *good night, sleep tight,* we know when it is time to transition despite objections from family and friends.

While experiencing the sinking feelings of helplessness along with depression, minds fade and people sleep more. When the end is near and people appear to be sleeping more, a dream state of heightened awareness may exist. This experience of Nirvana is the ability to be carefree, utilizing an injunction from the heart to *delete the need to understand.* With a clear mind and acceptance of death, we discover the heart's *healing presence* that allows for forgiveness. Like depression, to err is human, but depression triggers feelings of being unworthy, unreconciled, and lacking forgiveness. Nirvana is experienced through forgiveness. Arising from a higher power, the healing presence of forgiveness can lift us beyond depression and into enlightenment and acceptance. Ideally, we resolve to forgive illness and let go of the hostility inherent in hanging on to life.

I enlist my higher power through elevating the heart's stature as being "the Almighty" and omniscient. The intention of my Advance Care Directive is to not seek from others what I seek from myself. I recognize that God abides in my heart and that I need to circulate my uncertainties through this omniscient center. In listening to my heart, His ultimate plan and my next step enact a resolution. Giving up for the sake of giving up is one way to deal with depression. Turning matters over to the heart resolves to give up by letting go, transforming depression into acceptance, inspiration and deliverance.

PART V

...

Deliverance Through Advance Care Directives

WISH 30:

Neo-Life upon Crossing the Finish Line

I work in a hospital with a birthing center. One expectant mother arrives by ambulance as two others waddle through the emergency entrance. Adrenaline stimulates painful contractions with panic-laden exhilaration, deceleration and pursed-lip panting. The water breaks, the bubble bursts and the pregnant woman blurts out, "How soon can I have the epidural?" Come hell or high water, in one magnificent "Oh, my God!" the certainty of being right is in delivery of this new life. The promise of tomorrow bursts forth in a moment of *now* upon crossing the finish line.

Similar to labor and delivery, there is a moment when we might realize that death is imminent and declare, "It's time!" Swept up by powerful hormonal forces thrusting one into a tumultuous funnel of a birthing channel, this process leads to a new existence. Any sudden or crash landing requires bracing against impact by engaging in the chin-down, head-tucked, heart-focused position, a position assumed by an infant prior to the stork's landing. Ideally, the disaster victim and newborn emerge from their respective ordeals in the heads-up revelation of "I made it." While approaching death by negating or turning our backs, we assume the breech position of resistance rather than being fully engaged and forthright in a heavenly cause.

From the vantage point of pregnancy, the goal of Advance Care Directives is not to save lives in the womb of this world indefinitely, but to move through and beyond its passage when nature calls. Deliverance from the womb into the dawn of salvation is ours to imagine. The first trimester of advance care is wrought with anxiety over life's viability. Does the conception and diagnosis of terminal illness lead to new life or demise? Once the inevitability of death is determined, the second trimester affords palliative care as the fetus becomes jostled like a yo-yo through each stage of development. During the third trimester, the inherent struggle and ballooning burden feel as though something has to give.

Advance Care Directives are often written from the Yogi Berra perspective of *it ain't over 'til it's over.* Deliverance through Advance Care Directives freely proclaims, "I want this to be over." Perhaps we might agree to declare *it ain't over until the fat lady sings* . . . the so-called swan song. Similar to the swan being reluctant to herald its own impending death, the swan song of the dying is potentially buried deep and muted with a stiff upper lip. Deliverance becomes profound when those dying actually sing with contrition prior to death. We might confess to the deepest, darkest secret of actually being alien to this earth. Earth is a temporary assignment, not an everlasting home. My farewell confession and swan song emanates in *Jesu, Joy of Man's Desiring,* an unapologetic admission and expression of longing to return to a celestial bosom.

There is a time to live and a time to die. We might also embrace a desire to live and a desire to die. Desiring death appears treasonous to those left behind. We have a right to die, but others are reluctant to support the desire to break free of life. When the heart's desire is to die in peace, focus is directed toward fulfilling this promise.

While simultaneously conceding to death at the culmination of life, the threshold of an end zone comes into focus. Spectators might hail, "TOUCHDOWN!" A fumble in this end zone would feel like *dead man walking.* Deliverance seized in the end zone allows the receiver to triumphantly walk in the light. Final moments are given to gather thoughts and reflect on life with the prospect of having manifested the glory of God. From this position of certainty, the football is kicked with willpower and spirals absolute wholeness through the pearly goalposts of Heaven.

Advance Care Directives connote advancing to the very end. Crossing the finish line can only truly be attained upon death. Distinguishing the finish line from actual death creates time and space to honor the time to die through offering absolute freedom. People rarely allot time and space for goodness to flow from the end zone near death. Agreeing to receive advance care comes with a caveat of a breaking point, recognizing the demarcation between saving a life and honoring deliverance. Breaking this barrier to death requires breaking down entitlements that prolong life. Life has value. Does this demand entitlement to every measure that might sustain life? Spiritually, more is gained by keeping life and the end of life simple.

Recently, I returned from Hawaii and came to the realization that life is too short not to spend more time in Hawaii. What is ingrained at an early age is that life takes work. What I hear from retired people is they are busier now than while working. The need for speed and to succeed comes from the belief we never have enough, potentially making us gluttons for punishment. Maya Angelou poignantly stated, "There is a very fine line between loving life and being greedy for it." At the end of life, I aspire not to have more days, but to have more days with Hawaiian breezes. By nature, life is terminal. I see no reason to prolong life when illness creates more suffering. Deliverance from advance care replaces both the need for greed and intervention with relaxation and peace.

The desire to die is a different mindset. The barrier between saving life and accepting death could be similar to guarding one's virginity or enjoying sex. Letting one's guard down and engaging in sexual intercourse fully manifests the divine nature of procreation, circulation and makes the world go round. Through the conflicted martyrdom and merriment of lovemaking, fulfillment is eventually achieved with the afterglow of deliverance. The peak of human existence culminates in joy that exists following a robust sense of accomplishment. Joy arises from gladness, acceptance, and surrender, which are necessary feelings that allow for graceful transitions.

La petite mort, or "a little death," is French for orgasm. The ultimate orgasm in life is death. The antithesis of life being a blessing becomes realized as death being the ultimate blessing. Delaying orgasm during the heightened experience of living and averting coitus interruptus is naturally expected and encouraged. Most wish to enjoy the ride a little longer while others prefer it end sooner. Oddly, divine nature appears to be in conflict with cultural stipulations that resist any form of deliverance.

Equating the process of dying to having sex implies carefree abandonment prior to reaching ecstasy. When women die during childbirth, they never experience the ecstasy of holding their newborn. Many people die in the ED without having held a sacred moment for deliverance following the gestation of terminal illness. People rarely die in a good space. This realization prompts me to encourage people to achieve climax, let go and enjoy the aftermath of deliverance. Allowing the mind to transcend through the use of hallucinogenic or associative drugs might even enhance deliverance. Drug usage is generally considered bad behavior. Nevertheless, people who experience dementia and behave badly are justifiably medicated. If behavior is appropriate, there should still be nothing wrong with allowing people to get high in order to induce tranquility and achieve deliverance.

Tweeking is taboo when a person is considered self-respecting and health conscious. During deliverance, I intend to break from previous ways of thinking and behavior, perhaps indulging in the use of forbidden herbs and medicinal pleasures that release inhibition. As my spirit will eventually leave my body, why not skydive with an occasional out-of-body experience? This might be the best time to consider experimenting in life before becoming enrolled in a medical scientific experiment. To everything there is a season and a time to emerge from a cocoon. The new paradigm for a time to die might be deliverance to hasten death or "go fast" in a carefree state of wild abandonment. This fanciful "la-la land" potentially comes to light as the long-awaited Promised Land.

I often hear patients request, "Just knock me out," before beginning a procedure or an ordeal. In general, few physicians, faith-based families and communities or the healthcare system allow patients to break free and purposefully be knocked out. The Urban Dictionary provides several insightful passages as to what *knock yourself out* means. These include *going for it, going nuts; doing whatever the hell you want* or *working very hard to achieve a goal*. It is also noted that knocking yourself out suggests *incapacitating or rendering oneself unconscious by means of physical or mental abuse or deprivation of one's own body.[11]* I wonder if this would permit mercy killing. If incapacitated, I would anticipate ways to act out unconscionably and seize the day through nontraditional means.

I can only imagine what ecstasy feels like upon crossing the finish line or entering the end zone. The end of life might include a wish list for the last hurrah. Perhaps deliverance becomes the pivotal point of experiencing pleasure without an attachment to guilt. Deliverance might be considered waking on the last day of the rest of our lives, beginning the day with a super-sized cinnamon roll and a pound of bacon. While others might admonish us regarding personal end-of-life choices, we are all entitled to make the most of and not wallow in no-win situations. *If you got 'em, smoke 'em.* This is not the time to skimp on calories or skip dessert. *Last call* is an invitation for one final cocktail prior to *lights out*. This suggests contemplating closure before moving on to the after party or afterlife.

With respect given to being emancipated from being responsible, my father was free from dealing with overweight issues throughout his life. With confinement to a wheelchair and assisted-living, he has gained more than 40 pounds from eating institutional food. With his motto *to live and let die*, he now lives to eat and promotes his death with obesity. However, less responsibility and freedom has come with the sacrifice of no longer being able to smoke. Upon reaching the end zone of deliverance, I might consider smoking just to have the experience. Exhaling smoke rings might become provocative and exploitative in accepting death. While in the end zone, I wish to have enough time to enjoy more libation and liberty before death.

Individual bucket lists might include initiatives to pursue while healthy and indulgences to partake in when health is failing. Absolution of the need to be careful needs to aid the state of being carefree. The gravity of death allows for a shift in consciousness that defies being responsible and promotes being playful. I anticipate the prospect of retirement with each passing year and of what life experiences may remain on my bucket list. The end zone of life or time to die is a wonderful opportunity to experience life in an altered state of consciousness, doing those things we enjoy most while honoring those who bring joy to our lives.

WISH 31:

Neo-Logic for Integrating Good and Evil

I observe people at the end of life trapped in a state of repentance instead of celebration. They are consumed with thoughts of turning the clock back instead of enacting their last hurrahs. The idea of being carefree allows me to not work against dying. People often repent when disease is believed reversible and redeem wrongdoings in hope of living longer and being rewarded with a better afterlife. Deliverance is billed as the party to end all parties. My end-of-life directive would include pre-planning this celebration. During the time to die, my intention is to create a playlist of music and activities to nurture and reward my mind, body and spirit.

Deliverance from the usual way of thinking provides an alternative consciousness regarding redemption. Instead of achieving redemption by focusing on suffering, redemption might be perceived as living in a state of forgiveness. In pardoning ourselves, we are exonerated of shame and guilt, free to accept indulgences. As stated in the Lord's Prayer, I prefer that we *forgive us our trespasses as we forgive them* [illnesses] *that trespass against us,* forgiving any personal indiscretion that may have contributed to illness. Forgiveness of illness is rarely conceivable for people who believe death is undeserving. This lack of forgiveness is compounded by retaliation against illness rather than give peace a chance through acceptance.

Peace is often usurped when the end-of-life plan defaults to suicide. We tend to uphold and protect the sanctity of life while suicide remains a violation to the sanctity of life. Naturally, suicide is neither open for discussion—given the righteousness proclaimed in society—nor permitted in Advance Care Directives. However, when Advance Care Directives do not include an exit strategy, suicide is sometimes chosen as the only recourse. I worked with an ED registration clerk whose father committed suicide. There was no peace for her in this searing act of violence, and I doubt that he left this world in peace. Life can easily kill dreams. Attaining deliverance through the experience of dying can ensure sleeping forever in heavenly peace.

Peace can arise from the gift of atonement, being *at—one-ment* with good and evil. Perceived as God and Satan, these divine forces remain in perpetual conflict within each person. To live *rightly* compels us to reject and banish evil from our lives. Allowing for harmony and peace, good and evil are integrated by calling a truce between *healthy*—perceived as good—and *disease*—perceived as evil. Acknowledging that both deities contribute to the totality of divine nature provides deliverance. Illness is a necessary part of the totality of living. A wicked sense of humor actually permits the evil inherent to illness to actually be freeing. Through embracing the evil in divinity, reconciliation through the embodiment of deliverance does a body good.

Terminal illness undermines the hopes and dreams that are congruent with living. Reconciliation with end-stage disease provides an opportunity to kill illness with kindness. Illness is a natural predator to life and partnering illness with wellness creates the possibility of dying well. Averting the need to completely banish terminal disease allows for wholeness to simply be part of the game of life. Once and for all, the breeding ground of deliverance provides an invitation for the lion to lie down with the lamb. The image of these two natural enemies nestled together—free conflict—while creating peace. In the end, Advance Care Directives need to be explicit in allowing peace to flourish.

Wishes To Die For attempts to break down the barrier between good and evil, creating an acceptance of evil for the greater good. Dying rarely makes people feel like winners. The idea of a dying person as a loser needs to be changed to a dying person as a winner. *O' death, where is thy sting?* Aw, snap—Evil wins in the end. *O' grave, where is thy victory?* Good grief—winning occurs through the certainty of being right. Ultimately, feeling good about the inherent evil of illness rightly considers it to be rewarding. Illness is transformative and allows for each of us to feel blessed while transcending life. *Wishes To Die For* suggests unification rather than delineation of the virtues of good and evil.

A ruptured aneurysm creates a sentinel moment for a spiritual awakening. The same deliverance occurs through the process of dying. When dwelling on pain and suffering, people equate the idea of dying as evil. We are encouraged to live by the motto *what doesn't kill you makes you stronger,* but this can be amended to *what does kill you affords dignity* while providing a break from pain and suffering. Disrupting this paradigm of suffering averts the need to be stronger by proclaiming the certainty of being right with death.

My brother-in-law mentioned that his 82-year-old father with advanced Parkinson's disease developed pneumonia, sometimes referred to as the *old man's best friend.* The pneumonia had clogged a bronchus and collapsed a lung, creating respiratory distress. The doctor offered placing his father on life support. My brother-in-law justified the physician's offer by believing doctors are obliged to offer life-saving measures. His father could no longer eat and was emaciated. There are never any *have-to's* when patients are allowed to be carefree.

Dignity becomes risky business when patients wait too long to seek deliverance, becoming caught up in deliberation instead of liberation. With deliverance at hand, salvation could be gained either through the divine hand or by taking matters into one's own hand. Personally, I ascribe to the theological belief that *God helps those who help themselves.* My salvation does not come from God, but through linking peace of mind to the certainty of being right, breaking free of doctors' obligations. I am receptive to advance care only to the extent it will sustain my quality of life and personal freedom. When quality of life does not provide liberty, no advance care is necessary. I would welcome my rite of passage. When the door to advance care closes, the window of deliverance opens to end-of-life care.

Having an acceptance of death lends itself to the passive statement, "Do whatever you have to do." In Part I. I mentioned a woman with colon cancer who accepted death along with everything else the doctors were offering. Acceptance with deliverance allows for a more active approach in doing less. In other words, *let go and let God.* My higher consciousness remains mindful that I am a spiritual being. Spiritually, I am reminded, *for dust thou art, and unto dust shalt thou return* (Genesis 3:19). Spiritual beings are devoid of ego. The concept of a person returning to dust implies becoming nothing and that our true composition is actually biochemical and impersonal. Out of the dust I have the creative potential to use what is impersonal within me as a means to lessen my ego and detach from this life.

I vividly remember a gentleman, Steven, in his early 60s who was rerouted from the radiation oncology department to the ED after preliminary X-rays revealed another lung mass. The intended radiation treatment was canceled given this new development. Steven was both frightened and heartbroken. His doting wife and daughters were at his side, deeply concerned and speechless. I sensed this man wished to be free from further intervention and treatment that had proven to be unsuccessful. Most Advance Care Directives are created to minimize suffering, but rarely permit deliverance from doing more to sustain life. I was compelled to offer Steven deliverance by inquiring, "Are you done?"

Out of the depths of misery, Steven courageously declared, "I'm done." While family members cried, this patient gave a bittersweet verdict rendered with a sigh of relief. Steven's personal dignity seemed to beam in this moment of deliverance and certainty. Few of us are granted permission to walk in the light of deliverance, especially when neglecting to include a "get out of jail free card" within an Advance Care Directive. While Steven's death was certain, it was not imminent. In retrospect, I wonder if his deliverance was plagued by second guessing or flourished in triumph and ecstasy.

The relief that occurs in these situations and conversations is seismic, similar to when my patient, the Colonel, asserted his freedom and rights. Shedding end-of-life tears is followed by a sigh of relief. Through the release of both tears and suffering, deliverance is provided sooner rather than later. Advance Care Directives that do not allow for deliverance extend pain and suffering while prolonging life. The sooner the beginning of the end is appreciated as recorded in Advance Care Directives, the more time there is to flourish in the state of deliverance.

WISH 32:

Neo-Realization of Death as a Blessing

Physicians often fail to treat patients with dignity when family members figuratively tie their hands. Any appeal from a patient to "Let me go" needs to be adjudicated through a family conference, since such an appeal is typically not outlined in Advance Care Directives. Most directives express what may or may not be done medically, but rarely declare when people actually deem being done with life. The purpose of Advance Care Directives is not to ensure more care, but to declare how care is to be provided in order to grant a peaceful blessing at end of life.

I approached a daughter about deferring any further testing on her mother who was not long for this world. "I'm not ready to let my mother go," she responded. It became clear that I was no longer caring for the mother; now I was caring for the daughter. She managed to find the soft spot of my *wounded child*. I ordered the unnecessary interventions that temporally sustained her mother's life. Breaking the barrier between life and death is no simple task when there are ties that bind. Attention needs to be given to cutting the familial umbilical cord, permitting the realization of deliverance. What I confront most often in these situations is the age-old injunction, *What therefore God hath joined together, let no man* [or physician] *put asunder* (Mark 10:9).

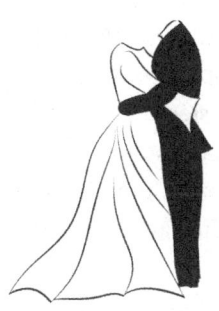

Advance Care Directives afford the opportunity to get all our ducks in a row. It becomes a personal duty to imprint the notion of dignity on the minds of family members who act as caregivers. Family members remain vigilant in looking for some sign or final word that imparts the certainty of being right with death. As patients receive the proverbial kiss of death, deliverance allows for this kiss to be transformed into a kiss of peace and be planted upon the foreheads of caregivers. All too often I observe patients detained in the Emergency Department until this final peace is rendered. When the intention is dying in peace, protection from harm begins by extending peace to those who potentially endanger dignity.

When considering the peaceful prospect of a so-called *good death*, the starting point is to consider death a blessing while having invoked God's favor. Naturally, to believe otherwise or to feel cursed provokes the idea of having a wrongful death. When personal freedom is increasingly compromised by illness, death could be easily appreciated as the ultimate favor. Consequently, death can be viewed from the perspective of being favored and chosen by God. Deliverance compels the gates of Heaven to swing open widely to a *good death*. Accepting death as a blessing extends peace to all around and furthers the realization of a *good death* as being a blessed one.

I often overhear people saying at funerals, "It's a blessing." This assumes that the deceased suffered hardship prior to death. When Advance Care Directives are written in an attempt to disallow death, there is little space for deliverance from hardship. The distinction between Advance Care Directives and end-of-life wishes occurs when life becomes less a blessing and death seems more appealing. Physicians are not trained to view death as a blessing and are therefore less likely to assist in making the end of life sacred.

Deliverance through Advance Care Directives allows viewing the end of life from the perspective of a beginner's mind, or a newborn baby. The expression "let sleeping babies lie" provides narrative to allowing nature to take its course in providing care to those dying. Creating distance between family members and the dying is analogous to protecting newborns in the sanctuary of a hospital nursery. From the window of the newborn nursery, loved ones can project their hopes and promises onto their babies, but with the imposition of a hands-off awareness. Boundaries allow for both newborn and dying having their individual journeys respected as life unfolds.

In the state of deliverance, patients become dissociated, distracted and childlike. Typically, children do not specifically communicate what is wrong or are aware of their wishes. Facial expression offers some indication of pain children experience. A child's breathing rate and chest movement/retraction provides an awareness of any distress. Pinching a child's nail bed and watching it pink-up is an indication of adequate blood flow. Healthcare providers actually surmise a child's wellness without the child saying a word or undergoing tests. At the end of life, I wish to be treated with the same respect healthcare providers give to children by not frightening them with intervention. Deliverance offers this prospective hands-off approach.

When it is clear the patient cannot be saved during an emergency situation, consideration is given to withdrawing medical care. The cardiac monitor is disconnected, medication infusion is discontinued and the patient might be moved to a less-equipped room in a less stressful environment. Family members take the place of healthcare providers at the bedside. This hallowed period of respite becomes ceremonial for providing unadulterated dignity to the dying person. Sadly, I rarely witness this time and blessing being given to patients when the tide rises to doing more to sustain life, dousing any prospect of dying with dignity.

The yin and yang of Advance Care Directives balance both active and passive, masculine and feminine energies. Advance care begins with aggressive treatment and ends with peaceful transition; from the yang state of being manipulated like a robot to the yin state of letting go like a rag doll. Consequently, *Dr. Yang* is necessary during the initial phase of terminal illness treatment, along with the support of *Nurse Yin*. Near the end of terminal illness, *Nurse Yin* takes the lead in providing the essential gifts of nurturing and receptivity that afford deliverance. The certainty of being right and feeling blessed transpires for the person while melting like a rag doll in the arms of the beloved.

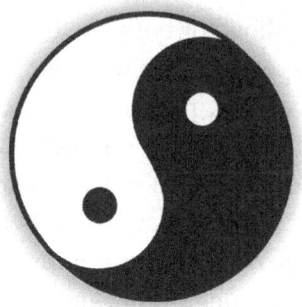

When a woman prefers natural childbirth, a physician's presence is unnecessary. This analogy holds true for patients wishing to die of natural causes. Dismissing a physician at the end of life might be perceived as either frightening or relieving. The dignity provided through deliverance becomes a blessing when a person is no longer realized as being a patient under a physician's care. There is no dignity in being a patient. Dignity is aligned with the certainty and desirability of being treated humanely through the natural process of dying. Theoretically, dignity potentially releases a physician's liability as patients assume more responsibility in preparation for death. Deliverance through Advance Care Directives shifts the paradigm of physicians from bedside to sideline.

When a physician dictates every aspect of end-of-life care, a conflict of interest is encountered. Typically, physicians fight disease while not giving up on patients. Generally, it is understood that a primary care physician steps aside when care is beyond the physician's level of expertise—an obstetrician provides prenatal care, a nephrologist provides care to a dialysis patient and an oncologist provides care to a cancer patient. However, patients tend to resist casually letting go of the seemingly important relationship with their primary doctor. When advance medical care appears to not be a viable option, receiving most physician care is no longer necessary or advantageous for patients.

The Norman Rockwell-like image of a doctor simply doing nothing other than holding a dying patient's hand or perhaps participating in patient-assisted suicide contradicts what most doctors believe to be right. The more patients are receptive to death, the less necessary it is for doctors to provide life-sustaining measures. When attention is called to a time to die through deliverance, advance care is unnecessary. However, few think physician care is unnecessary. When choosing to be treated humanely at the end of life, we need to concede remaining a physician's patient and reassert being human. Respect is given to human beings and rarely to patients. The novel idea of treating patients as human at the end of life requires a paradigm shift with a new care initiative. I title this "Omega Care."

WISH 33:

Neo-Concept of Omega Care

Just as life begins, progresses and ends—healthcare commences, advances and ceases to be effective. There are limits to what physicians within the present healthcare system can do to sustain life. Ideally, we have personal wishes to limit the means by which physicians are allowed to keep us alive. As people reach the point of not improving, they still often verbalize wishing to proceed with advance care. If not now, then when does the shift occur in receiving advance care to accepting death? When life becomes hopeless and death imminent, Omega care or end-of-life care potentially offers an olive branch.

Omega care might be considered hospice care that confers the blessing of deliverance. Hospice care in its hospitality strives to be all things to all people. In providing options for advance, palliative and end-of-life care, hospice care often provides confusion and uncertainty. I continue to manage hospice patients in the acute-care setting of the ED who have inappropriately presented for advance care. I recently cared for a female patient receiving hospice care whose death was imminent. Her family insisted on further evaluation and rehydration for relocation from Phoenix to Tucson. This woman was in transition, but not to Tucson.

In the past, hospice care honored the time to die. Presently, I believe hospice care leaves something to be desired. While advertising and promoting initiatives that encourage patients to live with more hope than humility, it has become a $17-billion industry. In addition, I currently find little distinction between hospice and palliative care. Palliative care emerged from hospice care with the goal of alleviating pain and suffering to provide better quality of life. Hospice care formerly offered palliation without curative intent, but this is no longer the case. While remaining focused on quality of life, hospice care potentially provides less dignity for the time to die.

Renaming hospice care to Omega care provides the distinct foundation for deliverance. End of life through deliverance empowers self-selection, less expenditure and a reprieve from enduring more suffering. Hospice care is generally what people make of it. Omega care is envisioned to be finite in loving people to death. Both palliative and hospice care continually offer confusing and coercive choices to patients promoting the idea that prolonging life is admirable. Mercy is the only admirable choice that would be provided by Omega care. In a directive to *choose this, not that,* I offer a side-by-side comparison of hospice and Omega care.

HOSPICE CARE	OMEGA CARE
Affirms Life	Affirms Rite of Passage
Hope Lingers in Limbo	Hope Dissipates through Bliss
Open-Ended Wishes	End-of-Life Wishes
Create Confusion	Create Certainty
Patient-Focused Care	Person-Focused Care
Monitoring Vital Signs –	Dismissing Vital Signs —
Objective Care	Subjective Care
Curative Care Optional	Curative Care Unnecessary
Intervention as Necessary	Rest in Peace
Physician Primary	Nurse Primary
Nurse Supportive	Physician Supportive
Compassion Needs Informed	Compassion Understood
Consent	Intuitively
Halfhearted Passive Euthanasia	Heartfelt Passive Euthanasia
Fear in Administering Mercy	No Fear in Administering Mercy
Queries Meaningful Life	Honors Fulfilled Life

Gaining any degree of control over destiny is empowering. Having personal dignity would assign certainty to the time to die. I listened intently while George H. W. Bush was struggling to recover from pneumonia. After being hospitalized for a month, he was moved to the Intensive Care Unit. As President of the United States he was considered the most powerful man in the free world; now his closest advisers were physicians. While rumors of his demise were greatly exaggerated, the president's situation reminded me of my father's situation: both men use wheelchairs and seem disengaged. The further I may become detached from life, the more I would prefer Omega care instead of intensive care.

A comparison can be made between living life and making love. The culminating peak of physical and emotional sexual excitement is referred to as the Big O, or orgasm. Extrapolating from this analogy, the Big O might be expressed as Omega. When life peaks and patients no longer respond to stimulation or treatment, they enter a refractory period. Any attempt at stimulating the body's nerves, muscles or organs is met with resistance and ultimately proves unsuccessful. Typically, the refractory period after an orgasm is brief. At the end of life this would be considered deliverance, with Omega care being provided. The certainty of being right with the Big O allows life to segue into a deep, permanent sleep.

Terminologies like "Omega," "Big O" and "refractory period" create a new appreciation for the time to die as crossing the finish line, enjoying the afterglow of fulfillment. Following orgasm, many people believe dying in that moment would mean dying happily. The contentment of life experienced during the refractory period is the virtual *pause, center and shift* from wanting more to drifting off to sleep. During this refractory period, patients often are recalcitrant or difficult to manage until they have resolved a simultaneous dilemma: Do they long to be left alone or "caressed" by medical therapy? Many patients find themselves in the ED during the protracted state of confusion that exists between a recovery lapse and a terminal refractory period.

A National Public Radio program comparing the post-sex behavior of introverts and extroverts intrigued me. Specifically, it addressed which of these two groups might prefer to cuddle after sex. After having sexual relations, introverts tend to rollover, detach from partners and drift off to sleep. Extroverts continue to remain engaged with partners following sex, postponing sleep. Palliative care might appeal to extroverts who long to cuddle on the deathbed. For introverts, Omega care might be the definitive way to post the *do not disturb* sign and signal being done. When duty ceases—both after sex and at the end of life—as an introvert I personally no longer wish to be engaged, coaxed or cuddled.

Many patients prefer to remain involved in the decision-making process of treatment. However, the wishy-washy nature of palliative care creates a type of limbo or purgatory. Palliative care provides plenty of space for patients to receive both aggressive and comfort care. This open-ended consideration for care has the potential to offer less certainty, depending upon who is caring for the patient and what the situation demands. There is always confusion between wishing that nothing further be done while continuing to seek additional medical care. Patients enrolled in palliative care tend to have fewer repeated trips to the Emergency Department. Omega care comes with permission to totally stop the revolving door of the ED. Omega care encourages contentment alongside potentially administering the last rites with a final blessing.

What seems awkward—and perhaps abusive—in the delivery of healthcare is waking patients to inform them that they are dying and need to have tubes shoved into their throats, stomachs or bladders. Furthermore, patients are forced to understand that this is being done to save their lives. Generally, these less-than-enthusiastic patients have little resistance and strength to object to such life-prolonging intervention. Dying patients risk sleep deprivation, perhaps becoming more careless than carefree. Palliative care allows patients to be enrolled in making choices. Omega care only allows for mercy and comfort.

Omega care is basically synonymous with comfort care. However, comfort care can imply comforting patients through ensuring everything be done to maximize the number of remaining days. Omega care would allow a person to die in peace rather than oblige standard medical practice. A physician's best practice is not withholding care that would allow illness to actually shorten a patient's life. Through accepting death and resigning to deliverance, patients might gladly accept their physician's resignation. Omega care is finite, becoming a means to an end through personal empowerment versus physician involvement.

Nurses or actual death midwives would provide the comfort care envisioned in Omega care. The focus of care moves from acute care to tender loving care, and from potentially beating people to death to loving them to death. This care might be considered negligent or passive, yet would be completely appropriate when patients desire a peaceful end-of-life transition. When the readiness and willingness to die exist, Omega care offers respect for this mindset. The patient would not be repeatedly questioned to death about further choices regarding treatment. Omega care presents patients with a *Do Not Disturb* sign.

WISH 34:

Neo-Alignment of Directives with Desires

Another way to think about Omega care is expelling the need to see and chart numbers. Most patients prefer to be treated as persons rather than numbers. However, the healthcare system is fixated on tracking and improving numbers. Most people can typically sense when a person is near death and rarely need to feel for a pulse in order to determine the gravity of the situation.

We are conditioned as patients to hold out our arms for vital signs to be taken, blood to be drawn and injections given. Meanwhile, people gaze at monitors and wonder what all the numbers mean. Numbers are irrelevant to those dying. Emphasis is better directed toward how patients feel. As patients, do we let go of objective numbers that suggest life is winding down while elevating the prospect of being cared for subjectively? Omega care provides people the option to be treated personally rather than objectively; not as a number, but with an abundance of tender loving care, appreciation and affirmation.

More important than the order *Do Not Resuscitate* would be to boost its understanding to mean *No CPR (No Check Pulse Rate)*. Patients are connected to machines that monitor vital signs with alarms that sound precipitate ongoing medical action. When patients prefer to rest in peace, monitors that impose calls to action interrupt peace. Ideally, less intervention results when vital signs are no longer taken. Caring less about blood pressure and oxygen saturation implies the readiness to die. Patients might politely remind family members to shift their focus away from numbers and care more about them as persons. When deliverance beckons, the first order of Omega care is to cease and desist from checking vital signs.

A patient receiving hospice care is not obliged to sign a DNR. Without this signed document, hospice care continues to permit resuscitating patients over providing dignity. Some people seemingly perceive signing a DNR as selling their souls to the devil, risking eternal condemnation. Omega care would be all-inclusive and honor the time to die without requiring informed consent or having people feel like they were signing their life away. With no attention given to checking vital signs in Omega care, resuscitation orders would be automatically rescinded.

Unlike hospice care, Omega care would have a standing order for DNR. It makes sense that end-of-life care necessitates a DNR. In the present healthcare system, a DNR order actually confuses healthcare providers, patients and family members. A DNR seems to imply and include the preference for patients to not be treated with heroic measures. However, a DNR only means patients do not wish to be resuscitated when their hearts stop. They may actually prefer to be treated with heroic measures up to that point and remain open to any and all potentially inappropriate medical intervention prior to death. I consider these patients to still be receiving palliative care.

Advance care planning is allows patients to maintain a "pulse" on their medical situation and prognoses. Reasonable people with poor prognoses express and demonstrate their personal characters through enlisting or averting heroic measures as documented in their Advance Care Directives. Medical prognoses provide the impulse and rationality for specific care.

End-of-life care can be divided into four *Pulse Options:*

1. I wish *everything* be done to sustain my pulse — Advance care.
2. I wish *some things* be done to sustain my pulse — Palliative care.
3. I wish *nothing* be done to sustain my pulse — Omega care.
4. I wish *nothing* be done when my pulse ceases — Definitive care (DNR).

When all that is truly desired is to be comfortable at the end of life, hospice care is considered. However, I rarely witness hospice patients being made comfortable in the ED setting. Omega care can afford patients the real opportunity to be excused from receiving more acute-care measures and needing to reiterate the heart's desires each time situations become worse.

The Pulse Options redefined from the perspective of dignity allow Advance Care Directives that provide more direction and certainty:

1. Advance care provides the certainty of being right by having all heroic measures implemented even with end-stage disease. The physician remains totally engaged while treating the illness aggressively.
2. Palliative care provides less certainty of being right. Patients neither hasten nor postpone death during end-stage disease. The physician offers conservative treatment.
3. Omega care provides the certainty of being right with total respect given to the dying. The physician is supportive of compassionate care provided by nurses.
4. Definitive care provides the certainty of being right determined by fate. Patients dismiss the right to die while leaving it up to a higher power. Healthcare providers stand down at the time of death.

Healthcare decisions usually depend on the circumstance and patient's level of competency. I am unable to anticipate my level of competency from one day to the next or what circumstance I might face. However, my level of competency would determine and dictate the care I wish to receive, as noted in my Advance Care Directive and attached Affidavit for Passive Euthanasia (Will to Die):

1. Advance care is my directive if I am deemed fully competent.
2. Palliative care is my directive if I am deemed partially competent.
3. Omega care is my directive if I am deemed incompetent.
4. Definitive care is my directive if I am deemed indifferent.

Typically, heart rates slow down toward the end of life. Are Advance Care Directives created to trust personal intuition arising from the heart that seeks to slow down or stop, as in Pulse Options 3 and 4? Or is the heart rallied to resume beating as in Pulse Options 1 and 2? When terminal illness is fully accepted as being terminal, an empowering directive permits the heart to expire.

Spiritually, the arms and hands are considered an extension of the heart. Trust arises from the heart. The desires of our hearts are entrusted and enlisted through Advance Care Directives by our own hands. Deferring care to the pulse generated by the heart essentially places end-of-life care in the "hands" of the heart. Naturally, peace of mind arises from trusting the heart rather than acting against it and creating more suffering.

Pulse Options 1 and 2 take full advantage of medical intervention to sustain life. Pulse Options 3 and 4 respect natural death. In the Emergency Department, most patients seek care that is consistent with advance and palliative care. The directive for Omega care is to offer more of a commonsense approach to end-of-life care and aligns the certainty of being right with common sense. This is deemed passive or voluntary euthanasia—supporting a will to die but not a blatant lethal injection. Omega care supports the patient's ultimate wish and heart's desire to die gracefully.

WISH 35:

Neo-Conservative Non-verbal Compassion

End-of-life conversation is difficult, but it can be exciting and enlightening when compared to retirement. For those who intend to work until they die, advance care is presumed undertaken as a type of directive. For those choosing semi-retirement while working part time, palliative care might be the preference. Those who intend to retire completely might eagerly become enthralled with Omega care. It concerns me when people are coerced into receiving a particular care plan that is incongruent with their retirement plan. As I envision becoming semi-retired and eventually needing to live semi-independently, I understand palliative care is called for upon reaching this stage in life. When I can no longer live semi-independently, I will seek Omega care. Most people who retire anticipate having less stressful lives and their care directives need to evolve and reflect their change in lifestyle.

No stagnant healthcare directive can adequately address the needs of a terminally ill patient. The Advance Care Directive needs to evolve as a patient's situation deteriorates. As opposed to what the Advance Care Directive may state, there is no ethical reason to flood a patient with antibiotics and blood transfusions when the situation is futile. There is always considerable confusion between sustaining life and providing comfort. Antibiotics and blood transfusions have potential side effects that potentiate suffering. The real intention of Advance Care Directives is to promote common sense, not to prolong pain and suffering.

My common sense was challenged by the passionate elderly wife of a senile patient who required additional blood transfusions for ongoing bleeding from an inoperable colon tumor. He had been returning anemic and weak to the ED on a weekly basis. I strongly felt that consideration was needed to responsibly end this irrational situation. Personally,

I was certain I would prefer to die from weakness rather than experience locked bowels caused by a growing tumor. Applying the survival rule of three, I suggested she might consider her husband receive three additional transfusions and allow nature to take its course. In retrospect, who am I to impose on others what is empathetic and ethically right? There are moments like these when I wonder if I cross the line.

Curiosity swirls around the issue of empathy being paramount to providing end of life. This becomes heightened as people rubberneck around the closed curtain in the ED. Behind the curtain is there a dead body, trauma patient or a routine ED diagnostic visit? Curiosity causes people's antennae to be raised, tuning into whether they can help the situation or wondering if the physician is responding with empathy. Upon entering a patient's room, I immediately determine whether I will be able to save the patient or if the situation is beyond my capacity. Generally, I encounter family members less interested in what I may believe would be empathetic and simply prefer I go about my business of saving the patient. When I hear concerns that doctors are not empathetic, I wonder why more attention is not given to what physicians feel is right for patients.

The conflict patients confront at the end of life is appearing weak when succumbing to illness. Most equate dignity with being strong-willed and tend to resist death and dying. This hotspot reminds me of a hot yoga class that sent up a red flare. During the practice, the instructor compassionately asked if anyone was feeling too hot. I remember thinking that if you need to ask, then it must be too hot. This question disturbed me because it sounded as though the instructor was daring the profusely sweating students to declare being weak. Naturally, the die-hard students were reluctant to demonstrate weakness. Similarly and empathically, is it necessary to ask a suffering patient if they need their pain relieved?

A compassionate care provider knows there is no need to ask heated, highly charged questions in a no-win situation. A gut feeling and empathetic response silences questions regarding life support. People long for someone to turn down the heat at the end of life without having to surrender and declare being weak. Naturally, empathy with compassion takes the expectation out of end-of-life choices. Ideally, we might waive our rights to informed consent and perhaps even decline listening to any bad news that requires making further choices. Ultimate freedom lies in being free from having to make further decisions. While enrolled in Omega care, the decision has been made once and for all with the understanding to please *turn down the heat*.

Good conscience and human nature are in conflict when challenged to have empathy for or provide compassion to people who lack common sense. Health providers and caregivers are no exception. Patients with no compassion toward themselves rarely elicit compassion from others. Patients tend to lack compassion when receiving poor prognoses and exhibit poor judgment. When compassion is a goal at the end of life, what is achieved and what is received might be the cruel and unusual punishment incited by the sentiment, "It is time for you to go." When patients and family members insist on advance care in lieu of the more compassionate Omega care, let them beware of *suffering sassafras*.

Omega care is congruent with my plan to board a virtual cruise ship at the end of life. Palliative care would require staying close to home with a hospital nearby. Palliative care affords options that address potential heart attack, stroke or pneumonia. In the concept of Omega care, these events would be viewed as precursors to death. Physicians inform patients who are receiving palliative of their options while patients enrolled in Omega care inform physicians that their services are no longer needed. Omega care would allow people a restful sleep. While asleep, most people do not concern themselves with needing hydration, nutrition and medication. The ideal prescription for better sleep at the end of life is provided through Omega care.

Omega care as passive euthanasia serves to fill in the gap between loitering in hospice/palliative care and wishing for assisted suicide or active euthanasia. By my definition, Omega care would allow me to be unassisted and detached from life-sustaining measures. Ascribed in my present Advance Care Directive is the phrase: *This Declaration shall constitute clear and convincing evidence of my intent in all circumstances.* However, there is often no real clarity in end-of-life circumstances. Through deliverance, clear and convincing knowledge is that all paths lead to death. My preference is to have a clear path upholding death. As my getaway plan, Omega care would honor my desire to not be kept in the loop, hindered by further bad news and hanging on indefinitely.

I cannot expect anyone to respect my desire to rest peacefully at the end of life until I create appropriate boundaries that protect me from well-meaning family members, caregivers or healthcare providers. Personal time needs to be respected and balanced with family and friends wishing to gather at bedside. Healthcare providers understand the wishes of the patient as relayed by family members. However, patients need to keep a short leash on family members who are inclined to push for further intervention.

Omega care provides permission to put down the phone and defer calling 911. When a patient is expected to die, it still seems that someone dying at home is always considered an emergency. I expect my father will die soon. My mother will probably call 911 when he dies or is near death. Like most of us, my father will have very little say when he reaches this point. "Whatever Mother thinks" has always been his safe zone. Omega care would not only provide a true safe zone, but would also offer paramedics more clarity to better decide whether to intervene in the potential hysteria surrounding end of life. Paramedics might offer immediate comfort and passive attention to present caregivers rather than attempting to resuscitate the patient.

Some people joke about having "DNR" tattooed on their chests. Most have the desire for their end-of-life wishes to be boldly communicated and taken seriously. I welcome this level of in-your-face communication rather than needing to explore patients' wishes buried in the mound of blankets shielding them. I appreciate and respect people who prefer to keep wishes personal. However, I also appreciate my 86-year-old neighbor who is adamant about expressing her refusal of life-saving measures. She anticipates and readily communicates her concerns regarding possible misunderstanding and mistreatment if unable to speak.

Ideally, Advance Care Directives that mandate wishes would be readily available while enduring a terminal illness or when reaching a certain age. While wishing to die with the certainty of being right, people confusingly distribute copies of Advance Care Directives to healthcare proxies, primary care physicians, hospital medical records, safe deposit boxes and online state registries. Interestingly, only 30 percent of people have Advance Care Directives, and the whereabouts of these tend to be left to the imagination. People often die suddenly and end-of-life wishes need as much visibility as medic alert bracelets. I propose people who value their wishes wear an end–of-life decision band, particularly while receiving palliative care.

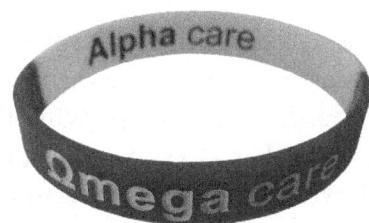

A neon wristband allows people to boldly communicate end-of-life intentions and care, forcing acknowledgement of their choices. Dignity does not add to the certainty of being right when people are not open to discussing death. Expressing their acceptance of death motivates those genuinely seeking dignity while dying. As a physician, I look for any sign that indicates a patient's desire to *do or die*.

I prefer not to give an impression of being insensitive to any wish that prolongs life when a patient appears to be dying but is not ready to die. I am sensitive to my patient's dignity being compromised if I am coerced into providing aggressive treatment when death is imminent. Compassionate and perceptive physicians notice nonverbal cues calling attention to matters of the heart, the dignity within the patient and the receptivity to accept death. Will this patient be comfortable with physicians providing less aggressive treatment, or will they perceive doing less as being uncaring? How are physicians to gauge a patient's receptivity to discuss this complex predicament and paradox? Dying with dignity is only realized through the empowerment attained from engagement.

Wearing the well-known Livestrong Foundation wristband sports the gauntlet of cancer survival. Similarly, wearing an end-of-life decision wristband makes a statement of individual freedom and empowerment with the directive that communicates personal authority over one's dignity. The original yellow Livestrong awareness band has morphed into every shade of color, promoting numerous organizations and causes. Building on its popularity and success, I designed an end-of-life decision wristband that communicates the ultimate choice to live or die. In support of a person's choice to live or die, the awareness band has two distinctive sides. One is a bright yellow, embossed with "Alpha care," while the other is a subdued blue, embossed with "Omega care." As with other awareness bands, the empowering Alpha care/Omega care decision wristbands display one's current wish to live or die.

This decision band serves as an emblem that promotes the cause and increases awareness regarding Omega care. While the Alpha care/Omega care decision band is neither a legal document nor an Advance Care Directive, it can be the voice for people unable to speak during the profound and decisive moment of potentially dying with dignity. It is a visual statement and the fundamental imperative distinguishing whether more or less care is provided at the end of life. Ultimately, the purpose of Omega care is to honor and grant peace through less intervention.

While placing importance on end-of-life wishes, it is odd that most Advance Care Directives are missing in action when patients present to the ED and directions are most needed. Being unprepared for death, family members are often reticent to be forthcoming with Advance Care Directives that support a patient's wish to die. Similar to Automated External Defibrillator (AED) chest pads that provide an immediate recognition of heart rhythm that determines intervention, Alpha care/Omega care wristbands provide a "quick look" regarding heartfelt wishes that deserve respect.

Marriage is considered one of the major decisions made in life, stating the vow "Until death us do part." A wedding ring shows that the individual is taken and connotes commitment and ownership of this decision and the relationship. However, the ultimate decision in life consciously determines the end of life. Dignity is expressed through taking personal ownership of the choice to live or die, proclaiming this boldly with an Alpha care/Omega care decision band and remaining true to there is *a time to live and a time to die.* The integrity of this choice is symbolic in the wristband and becomes more significant when the Omega care side is displayed, signifying the time to die. This becomes a statement regarding the certainty of being right with death.

Choosing to wear an Alpha care/Omega care wristband indicates the importance of dying with dignity to the individual. My concern in caring for patients with the certainty of being right would be alleviated through their wearing this wristband, averting treatment decisions made through insinuation or potentially insulting questions regarding minimizing patient care. The assumption is made in the current healthcare system that all patients prefer Alpha care unless otherwise indicated and documented. To opt out of this type of Alpha-care mentality, more choice and credence needs to be paid to Omega care.

Life-and-death choices incite similar arguments regarding pro-life and pro-choice in the abortion issue. I imagine people becoming polarized through self-determination and external demonstration of courageously displaying this Alpha care/ Omega care wristband. I anticipate hearing external debate that delves internally as the certainty of being right causes battle lines to be redrawn while individuals choose sides. People long for more control of decisions made on their behalf while receiving palliative care. During this time, the decision band becomes imperative for individuals to regain control. Realizing that life ends, Alpha care cannot be the end-all for patients who have aspirations to die with dignity. Displaying "Alpha care" on the decision band serves as a reminder to actively *pause, center and shift* with the knowledge that choice and control are synonymous with reversal of the band—displaying "Omega care" when the time feels right.

The Alpha care/Omega care wristband shines a light on dignity in the context of divinity with the proclamation: *I am the Alpha and the Omega; who is, who was and who is to come, the Almighty* (Rev. 22:13). The prospect of being deemed "almighty" at the end of life seems ludicrous. Nevertheless, proclaiming to be almighty and a force to be reckoned with is a wish to die for that the decision band supports. As Omega care advances the paradigm of patients having more control with less suffering, the Alpha care/Omega care decision band actually puts a welcomed spin on choice and responsibility regarding the adage: *you've made your bed, now lie in it.*

Life is a reality and death inevitable. Creating personal reality provides the opportunity and responsibility to choose a personal death and afterlife. Free choice is inalienable and creates personal power. Lives are spent making choices, rarely escaping the confrontation of death as a choice and remembering that not wishing to die is also a choice. Spirituality enlists the creativity that allows for choice. The creative energy swirling within the universe allows for certainty through divine intelligence and order. Armed with the potent gauntlet of the Alpha care/Omega care decision band, people would engage world order and purposefully enter the Promised Land.

WISH 36:

Neo-Horizon of a Promised Land

I never really know what lies behind the next curtain as I slide it open and greet the patient. I emphatically tell nurses not to spoil my surprise or say anything that might bias my objectivity. I walked behind the curtain one day and was pleasantly surprised by the radiance of a young woman experiencing lower abdominal pain. She exuded an unusual amount of confidence despite her pain and I could not help but ask, "What makes you smile?" She proudly expressed having lost 50 pounds and her determination to lose 20 more. Her response prompted me to think that significant weight loss might actually be experienced as losing a former self. The journey of weight loss and self-remodeling leads to having a different perspective of life while setting course to a better place or the Promised Land.

I observe this type of transformation in patients who have experienced heart attacks. Oftentimes these patients become mindful and begin to model eating healthy, exercising regularly, not smoking and taking medication as prescribed. The goal is not to have another heart attack and increase their chance for longevity. Being our best adds certainty to life's journey. Inasmuch, the journey to the Promised Land begins by following the yellow brick road of self-discovery. Certainty is perceived as reaching the Promised Land in the hope of having the Wizard of Oz grant a wish or blessing. Ultimately, reaching the Promised Land is achieved through the discovery of the wizard within along with the realization that having a brain, heart and courage is inherent and interconnected within each person.

The television show *Extreme Makeover: Home Edition* never fails to bring a tear to my eye as it tugs at my heart. In an appeal to the producers of the show, families provide compelling stories of having endured hardships while advocating their home be selected for a makeover. There is great anticipation in a new house having a positive impact on the family. Once chosen, the home is gutted and refurbished in a reflection of triumph over hardship. The family eventually returns home on a bus with blacked-out windows, proceeding to step outside. There is a call in unison to "Move that bus!" Suddenly, the great reveal and curb appeal of a new house and better life profoundly appears before their eyes. In reality and at the end of life, this bus would not be easily moved. We might need to move our eyes vertically and spiritually to see the Promised Land when obstacles present.

The TV show we all have the opportunity to star in might be referred to as "Extreme Makeover: Dying Edition." The process of dying changes people while opening up the prospect of receiving a *makeover*. Replacing the word "dying" with the word "makeover" immediately connotes a more positive image and outlook. People fear change, but are likely to channel this fear into excitement when change is perceived as a *makeover*. Might the perception of dying be changed from a sad saga to a happy ending? I am certain that we have the capacity to die well through feeling better about ourselves. This realization permits blossoming at the end through fulfillment, happiness and gratitude. Fulfillment allows rising above pain and suffering through appreciating the beauty of life.

As a child, one of my favorite books was *Black Beauty.*[12] The author, Anna Sewell, was an invalid and staunch advocate for animal welfare. Illustrating the hardships endured by Black Beauty, the moral of her book was to encourage people to treat animals with kindness and respect, not to marginalize them as proverbial black sheep. Similarly, the life lesson that applies to *Wishes To Die For* is to explore the romantic notion of personal beauty and likeability being maintained as the end of life approaches, regardless of becoming ill or an invalid.

The moral to the end-of-life story needs a romantic twist of self-discovery regarding dignity. People who thrive live with hearty appetites and create opportunities to celebrate and dance. As we age the *twist* evolves from doing the hustle to attempting the boogie and finding a groove. Earlier in life, energy is often invested in personal growth with an emphasis toward creating a better life and overcoming shortcomings. Later in life, I appreciate moving perceived deficits into the asset column. For me, reaching the end zone of the Promised Land will occur when personal achievement becomes less important than actually living with fulfillment.

When life is experienced as less than fulfilling, the prospect of dying with dignity becomes less likely. The certainty of finding fulfillment depends on reaching our own version of the Promised Land. As the existence of an afterlife is questioned, there is no doubt that the end of life is the culmination of fulfillment. I envision both fulfillment and the Promised Land being cultivated by stewardship through responsible planning and management of resources. Similar to stewardship, there is the capacity to plant seeds and reap what is sown. In the Promised Land field of dreams, having dignity potentially allows people to flourish at the end of life.

The Promised Land is a place we can only imagine. It is a place beyond feeling held captive by disease or circumstances beyond control. In biblical terms, the Lord promised to lead the Israelites out of Egypt into the Promised Land flowing with milk and honey. This concept of paradise being the perfect place that allows for a blissful state of being is of our own making. If there were to be a remake of the film *It's a Wonderful Life,* might we shine in the leading role? This type of imaginative thinking offers the vantage point and foresight to view life as having been wonderful and deserving. I believe we all deserve a bountiful afterlife of whatever our hearts desire.

As the existence of Heaven is questionable, we still tend to collect images of the Promised Land, similar to amassing keepsakes proudly displayed as collections. As a young child I was encouraged to add jewels to the crown I hoped to receive upon entering Heaven. The brilliance of my life would be reflected in this crown. In the context of Catholic faith, my coronation would involve wearing this crown while seated next to God. Through the make-believe images created during childhood, most children imagine being king or queen and having rule over a presumed Promised Land or sovereign territory overflowing with riches.

End-of-life health issues have a way of stripping people of earthly regality, sovereignty or abundance. The parable of the rich man and Lazarus explains: *There was a rich man who dressed in purple garments and fine linen and dined sumptuously each day. And lying at his door was a poor man named Lazarus, covered with sores, who would gladly have eaten his fill of the scraps that fell from the rich man's table. Dogs even used to come and lick his sores. When the poor man died, he was carried away by angels to the bosom of Abraham. The rich man also died and was buried* (Luke 16.19-22). While patients, as beggars, cannot necessarily choose their afflictions, they can still choose to be among those carried off by angels. The exceptional patient, as the rich man, will feel indignation or forsaken.

Imagining a better place with more than enough of everything is contrary to the experience of being in an Emergency Department. When patients present to the ED, they generally lack the wherewithal or resources necessary to improve their medical ailments. Sometimes health providers meet patients' expectations, but I do not consider the ED being remotely close to the Promised Land. The aforementioned young woman with her aspiring self-confidence simply needed reassurance as to whether her pain was serious. She had pre-determined how she would handle her pain, enhancing the certainty and radiance that would naturally exist in the Promised Land. I wanted to bottle her energy and self-validation and share this nuance with others.

WISH 37:

Neo-Nuance of Self-Validation

I perceive the Promised Land as a place the heart longs to abide, personally realizing self-validation and worthiness. An intimate relationship often provides validation and affirmation, becoming jeopardized during the process of dying. Unfortunately, during the state of deliverance we are typically susceptible to experiencing self-deprecation and invalidation. Dignity provides the means to perceive and support the ability to self-validate "in spite of dungeon, fire and sword." This lyric from the hymn *Faith of our Fathers* reminds me that through faith, we might actualize a higher power of self-validation, supporting the certainty of being right. Ideally, *Wishes To Die For* promotes self-validation by cross-examining wishes.

On a personal level, I achieved deliverance when no longer wishing to be like everyone else and accepted my homosexuality. However, I initially needed to be delivered from having the perception that people would rather die than be gay. This reminds me of the ridicule I endured as a child when others taunted, "I'd rather be dead than red on the head." My certainty of being right collapsed upon the certainty of being wrong once I was perceived as different. Ironically, while becoming nearer to God to pray away the gay, I was befriended by several priests. My own "Book of Revelations" opened when one priest spoke of his boyfriend. I questioned why I had not received the memo that it was acceptable to have sex outside marriage, particularly with another man. Biblically speaking, God provides messages through "parables" defined as "a story designed to illustrate some truth, religion principle or moral lesson."[13]

As a gay man, I can testify that principles for *doing right* are generally heard from the outside and often directly conflict with the certainty of *being right* as heard from the inside. No one can determine another person's sexual orientation. Sexual preference arises from the self-awareness and discovery of what feels right. What feels right contributes to awareness, fueling acceptance and ultimately deliverance. This appreciation of an alternative way of thinking supports my alternative state of consciousness regarding death. My salvation will never occur through the feelings of others. Letting go of old thought patterns that no longer serve me well prevents suffering. I achieve the state of deliverance through self-validation.

In retrospect, I appreciate the halfhearted aspect of parental validation. The door my parents closed by not fully embracing my sexual orientation opened the window of possibility through self-validation. Thereby, I came to accept my sexual orientation as being truly wonderful through self-validation. Wishing to transform this relationship from judgment to heart-centered, I invited them to lunch. While seated across from my parents, I opened my heart with, "What makes my life wonderful is not being a doctor, but being your son and I'm here to thank you." Equivalent to the Berlin Wall tumbling down, this breakthrough moment allowed deliverance to be revealed and bestowed.

Upon further reflection, my life is not wonderful because I am a doctor, but because I am a gay man who appreciates and has mastered the art of self-validation. I may have missed this valuable life lesson had my parents previously validated me as being gay. An important insight highlighted by Dr. Joy during his Initiation into the Heart Center Conference was that children do not possess the ability to self-validate. Adults have the capability to self-validate, but this becomes a slippery slope when they prefer not growing up.

As we become elderly—and perhaps more childlike—the ability to self-validate wanes. In growing old gracefully, it becomes incumbent on us to retain self-validation. The key to accepting and honoring the passage of dying through the adversity of aging is interchanging self-validation and gratification. Fear of death never allows for gratification during the process of dying. Gratification is the source of pleasure or satisfaction that arises from the heart and remains important throughout the process of dying. Self-worth and gratification become realized with comfort in being alone with our selves. While dying, we need support from the heart in this endeavor.

WISH 38:

Neo-Insurgence of Resurrection

As actions speak louder than words, gifts from the heart leave us speechless. The true gift of life is personified as love in action. Using the right words in conjunction with an act of love is similar to expressing the sentiment attached to a gift. Advance Care Directives are typically written from the perspective of continued well-being and survival; deliverance from these directives expresses actions to be taken in consideration of others. In addition, we might *pause, center and shift* attention on Advance Care Directives from personal and self-centered to impersonal and heart-centered, honoring the heart's attribute of *unconditional love* during the time of deliverance.

My interpretation of deliverance originates from the example of Jesus Christ in His teaching, *The good shepherd lays down his life for the sheep* (John 10:11). A similar message of deliverance is found in those enlisting in military service and dying with honor in the cause of freedom. *The Battle Hymn of the Republic* artfully describes and conveys the end-of-life scenario between Christ and a soldier: "As He died to make men holy, let us die to make men free." The battle hymn of Advance Care Directives enlists battles that occur at the end of life, eventually surrendering lives in the cause of freedom. In honoring this unconditional cause, *There is no greater love than to lay down one's life for one's friends* (John 3:16).

Honoring the concept of deliverance and giving my life up for personal freedom may appear selfish or selfless. The journey to the Promised Land is paved with both integrity and receptivity; following through with intention and being willing, ready and open to wholeheartedly enter the Promised Land. The mechanics of the heart provide ongoing conscious examples of receptivity and acceptance. The heart receives what the veins provide without judgment. The mind is resistant to incoming information that threatens survival. I appreciate the conflicted struggle regarding deliverance in almost every yoga pose. I am prayer-fully reminded to quiet the mind and open the heart through a personal introspective mantra recited as:

Quiet, silence
Create stillness
Remain centered
Be receptive

Allowing receptivity through the heart relaxes mind and body. Receptivity is a type of "girl power" that allows for dancing—a creative playful flow of energy from one pose to another. Initially, being at ease with receptivity and femininity was challenged when I crept into an all-female yoga class. I needed to overcome the belief that I was going to die of embarrassment. People die all the time, usually with a sense of shame rather than receptivity. Receptivity is realized as a sponge that craves flexibility in completing a task. Yoga is described as a disciplined practice with one of its benefits being receptivity. Transformation occurs when continually showing up and practicing receptivity. As in deliverance, transformation through empowerment occurs through uniting masculine and feminine energies into one electrical charge.

Similar to flipping a light switch, the circuitry inherent to existence remains as unconscious as breathing. Yoga encourages being aware and remaining conscious of breathing. Deliberate breathing provides for the renewed consciousness of life. In deepening the breath and expanding lung capacity, less energy is expended and more awareness is given to enriching life. When breath quickens or is constricted, life is shortened. Life is the ongoing process of inhalation and exhalation—inhaling the acceptable and exhaling the unacceptable. Recognizing that breathing is unconditional to life and controllable, there is an appreciation of when inhalation is complete and when to let go.

The cyclic nature of life and death provides the never-ending awareness and opportunity to both acknowledge and let go. The ability to acknowledge and let go is how to effectively cope with life challenges. Coping might be best visualized as flushing the toilet. Shit happens—acknowledge it and flush it. After the toilet bowl refills, it is subjectively perceived as half-full or half-empty. Coping mechanisms typically play out as people deal with stressful situations by attempting to hang on or hang in there. People tend to hold their breath for fear of letting go. Coping is best achieved through remembering to breathe deliberately while repeatedly flushing the system. This primal force potentially eases stressful situations through intentional, optimistic visualization.

Inhalation is complete when fulfillment is experienced intuitively. When self-validation moves the conversation from *at least I have my health* to *at least I can still breathe*, breathing affirms life. Conscious breathing leads to the greater awareness of the meaning of life. This awareness spearheads my conclusion that all of life is a venture of personal fulfillment. Consciously accepting every breath allows for being receptive of life in this moment. In addition, to *pause, center and shift* with each inhalation is a means to achieve fulfillment. Believing everything happens for a reason, every moment becomes a blessing that potentially resuscitates a renewed inspiration to life through resurrection.

I visualized personal fulfillment through being seated at the window of an airplane prior to touch down. Transcendentally, I gazed at the beautiful sunset with a horizon flooded in glorious color. I perceived this as the splendor of my life. As the airplane's shadow came into view, I suddenly realized that it personified my own personal shadow. This personal shadow represented my ever-unconscious spirit destined to interface with my conscious mind upon impact with death. Before this moment, both plane and shadow ran parallel as two distinct forces, representing Air Force One and an accompanying fighter jet. Acting as the fighter jet, my unconscious spirit safeguards the dignity inherent to Air Force One, or the totality of my life that exists in the skies of the Promised Land and is now cleared for landing.

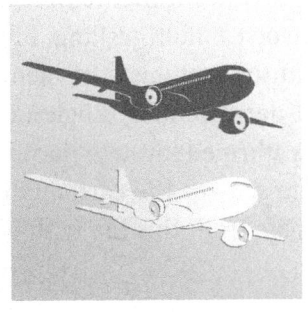

Union of the conscious and unconscious consistently occurs within the heart. While intimately connected with the soul, the heart would exchange messages with the mind. Within the center of existence between life and death, illness and healing, consciousness and unconsciousness remains a deeper mystery. In the gaping wound occurring from a life-threating illness, the mystery of healing is found in the soul. While attempts are being made to save the soul, the mind is left with a greater mystery of uncertainty regarding fulfillment. As such, Advance Care Directives originating solely from the mind tend to potentiate uncertainty. Advance Care Directives formulated in conjunction with the heart tend to honor the higher consciousness of the soul that grants certainty.

To die with a sense of fulfillment requires conscious effort. Unconscious forces that sabotage certainty compromise dignity. Similar to a dream state, these unconscious dynamics are likely to cause a startle response and ignite a wake-up call or call to action. When called to examine these unconscious thoughts and bring them into consciousness, the goal is to make sure our efforts support personal wishes. Unfulfilled wishes are a matter of personal responsibility. While dying, there is a tendency to maintain hopes and dreams for this life with the belief that it is never too late to have the life we desired. However, my Catholic upbringing inspires the concept of Resurrection—being able to rise above the passion and death contained within hopes and dreams in order to realize deliverance.

The glory of experiencing the Resurrection affirms life and is experienced in the celebration of Easter. Those living in the Resurrection are encouraged to say "yes" to whatever life offers while knowing full well that life gives and takes, builds and destroys. The ups and downs that affirm life actually create harmony. Typically, life is perceived as a linear process with a progressive incline, reminiscent of climbing uphill. However, life usually involves multi-tasking, linking both physical and spiritual inclinations with intonations. The blending of these tones and pitches, crescendos and decrescendos, single notes and chords, creates life's composition. Life is affirmed through harmony, creating tranquility.

The affirmation of life spawns the certainty of being right with the solemn declaration to pass from this life with dignity. The certainty of being right affirms life through honoring the circle of life that poten-tiates birth and rebirth, deliverance and salvation. Nurturing and af-firming life in concert with dignity is enhanced through the mirror of others doing right by us. Similar to the certainty of being right, quality of life is very personal and sets us apart from one another. However, the impersonal aspect of being separated from others is difficult to accept. Therefore, accepting the end zone of hospice care generally is in conflict with affirming life.

Nevertheless, hospice care supports and affirms quality of life by po-tentially providing unconditional love that is reinforced through Omega care. Deliverance is experienced when another provides unconditional love. When God's plan does not seem to include a miraculous recovery, miracles remain appreciated as extraordinary and transcendent bless-ings. The miracle provided through hospice care is deliverance found in the Promised Land. Like winning the lottery, a miracle is virtually impossible. However, I view hospice care, refined as Omega care, as be-queathing a jackpot of unconditional love to those dying.

Advance Care Directives that culminate in deliverance reassure fear with the passage, *Be still, and know that I am God* (Psalm 46:10). The heart offers *unconditional love* and this is the foundation of end-of-life care. Deliverance found in the Promised Land is a homecoming sur-rounded by unconditional love. Through a humble heart and the ex-ample of Lazarus, *it would come to pass, that the beggar died, and was carried by angels* [hospice] *into Abraham's bosom; the rich man died, and was buried.*

Wishes To Die For is essentially a scavenger hunt. We seek far and wide for the hidden treasure chest that is inherent and lies in the heart. Home is where the heart is, and the prevailing wish to die at home is more importantly realized as a wish to dwell amid unconditional love. This is the Holy Grail! Raised at the Last Supper, the Holy Grail was auspicious and symbolic of a *cup runneth over* of unconditional love. Deliverance through my Advance Care Directive will allow me to drink from this cup at my last supper. Hopefully, my last supper will be served in a place of safety, wonder, appreciation and love abiding in a spiritual realm recognized as *home*.

The scriptural depiction of unconditional love resounds in the passage that states: *For God so loved the world that He gave His only begotten Son, that whoever believes in Him shall not perish, but have eternal life* (John 3:16).[14] When God "gave" his Son's life in consideration of being the Sacrificial Lamb, was this blessing of euthanasia a blatant message that supports an example of unconditional love? Whoever abides in unconditional love "shall not perish" and potentially flourishes. People tend to perish when they hold onto life and create spiritual deaths, becoming poor souls. I witness spiritual deaths as heartbreaking and disconnected from the heart's desire. Only through physical death will staunch pro-life advocates attain eternal life.

Spiritual death occurs whenever remaining true to the heart is ignored. The perception of Advance Care Directives as spiritual documents encourages speculation about which actions lead to spiritual death or eternal life. Losing the game of life occurs while perishing and winning the game of life occurs through flourishing. With the mind-body disconnection that often occurs in the end zone, the ball is likely to be fumbled. Practice is needed in keeping the eye on the ball meant to land in sweet spot of the heart. Every trip to the Emergency Department is a reminder of human mortality. Every journey to heart-center is an acknowledgment that suffering related to mortality can be reconciled and resolved.

While fumbling for the "get out of jail free" card or the ticket to the Promised Land, many people will come up empty-handed. Many do not have this trump card stashed in their Advance Care Directives. Playing this trump card upon a sudden spiritual death raises awareness of winning the game after all by dying in peace. The spirit always gravitates toward peace, ultimately levitating from a deceased body. The spirit coaxes us to continually re-center and reaffirm life through connecting with peace, ultimately realized within the Promised Land.

I envision a ribbon cutting ceremony before entering the Promised Land. Generally, a person of authority or dignitary will cut the ribbon during the opening ceremony of a completed project. At this moment, passage is opened to the Promised Land. As the physician in charge and author of *Wishes To Die For*, I authorize the reader to become the supreme authority who cuts this figurative ribbon restricting access to the Promised Land. It becomes a personal responsibility to cut through manmade obstacles and transcend this life, similar to a releasing a balloon that will soar to infinity and beyond.

The end of life becomes a breakthrough moment of humanity and a *mea culpa,* my culpability. When acknowledging full responsibility for being human, acceptance of one's mortality is a call to die. Advance Care Directives afford the opportunity to choose end of life with the proposition *if you want something done right, do it yourself.* The certainty of being right maintains a conviction to personal integrity and responsibility. My dignity will be realized by responsibly doing it my way with the power vested in my heart.

The uncertainty that plagues death and dying is only reconciled through the heart. The certainty of honoring life pays tribute to the heart and generates gifts of gratitude, love and peace. Having said my peace and made my peace, *Wishes To Die For* is a gift of gratitude, labor of love, and invocation for peace. Peace arises from the sacred consciousness *to light and guard, to rule and guide* the end-of-life journey. Dying with dignity is an aspiration for sacred passage. The end-of-life journey as sacred passage embraces *compassion, innate harmony, healing presence* and *unconditional love*—securing each in the backpack of an Advance Care Directive.

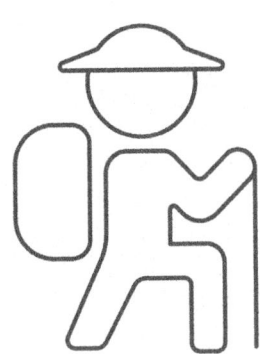

In homage to attributes of the heart carried in the journey of deliverance found in the Promised Land, I end with a stanza by A. E. Housman:[15]

> *Now hollow fires burn out to black*
> *and lights are fluttering low;*
> *Square your shoulders, lift your pack*
> *and leave your friends and go.*
> *O never fear, lads, naught's to dread,*
> *look not left nor right;*
> *In all the endless road you tread*
> *There's nothing but the night*
> [Amid the certainty of being right]

NOTES

1   Elisabeth Kubler-Ross, MD, *On Death and Dying* (New York: Scribner, 1969), 264.

2   Michael Armstrong, *Armstrong's Handbook of Management and Leadership, 3rd Edition* (Philadelphia: Kogan Page Limited, 2012), 306.

3   Don Miguel Ruiz, *The Four Agreements* (San Rafael, CA: Amber-Allen Publishing, 1997), 63.

4   Gale Sayers, *I Am Third* (New York: Penguin Group, 2001),viii.

5   Caroline Myss, *Anatomy of the Sprit* (New York: Crown Publishing Group, 1996), 40.

6   Robert Young, "Voluntary Euthanasia", Edward N. Zalta, ed. The Stanford Encyclopedia of Philosophy (Summer 2014 Edition) http://plato.stanford.edu/archives/sum2014/entries/euthanasia-voluntary/.

7   Neale Donald Walsch, *Conversations with God, Book 2* (Charlottesville, VA: Hampton Roads Publishing, 1997), 151.

8   Dean Koontz, *Fear Nothing* (New York: Bantam Books, 1998).

9   Gary Chapman, *The 5 Love Language* (Chicago: Moody Publishers, 2010), 191. To learn more about Gary Chapman and the love language concepts, and to discover your own primary language, visit www.5lovelanguage.com

10   Bob Lonsberry, *A Various Language* (Springville, UT: Cedar Fort, 2007), 169.

11   Aaron Peckman, *Urban Dictionary.com,* accessed July 19, 2012.

12   Anna Sewall, *Black Beauty* (New York: Barse & Hopkins), 1911.

13 All word definitions cited from Dictionary.com. *Dictionary.com Unabridged.* Random House, Inc.

14 All Bible scriptures cited from *The Holy Bible, New King James Version* (Nashville, TN: Thomas Nelson Publishers, 1982) and Donald Senior, ed. *The Catholic Bible Study—New American Bible* (New York: Oxford University Press, 1990).

15 Tom Burns Habor, The Manuscript Poems of A.E. Housman (Minneapolis, MN: Colwell Press, 1955), 17.

APPENDIX I

September 25, 2014

MY MOTHER, MARY

Being a child of God and having a mother named Mary has graced my life with divine relevance. My grade school. St. Mary's, bestowed honor on the sanctity of this name. Each May the prettiest girl in school crowned the statue of the Blessed Mother, Seemingly, a voice from Heaven had said to me, *This is My beloved Mary with whom I am well pleased* (Mathew 3:17). Eighty-eight years and counting, I am well-pleased to crown Mom's birth and her life. The double number 88 present the dual challenge and opportunity for the birthday girl to reign in splendor with self-mastery of her hopes and dreams.

My *mother of perpetual help* laid the foundation for me to be self-sufficient and conscientious. In wishing to emulate Mom, I fulfilled her aspirations of becoming a caring physician. In her self-proclaimed purpose to *do for others,* she became the ultimate caregiver/worrier. By repeatedly saying, "Everything has a place and there's a place for everything," she ensured that *orderliness is next to godliness.* With a resume that noted her being supervisor at every job she had while raising seven children, she has earned a seat next to God. In addition, the luck of the Irish promises her a pot of gold in Heaven, one overflowing from her generosity and sacrifices made while on Earth.

Her middle name, Anastasia, was the stone that her "builder" rejected. This represented the life she was given but never wanted. At age 88, will self-mastery allow the enchanting name of Anastasia to become the cornerstone that fortifies and supports her life as awesome? Anastasia means *Resurrection.* Each birthday presents an opportunity to be born again from a new vantage point. With age, birthdays are less about excitement and more about thankfulness. Excitedly, I use this occasion to pay homage and thanksgiving to her adorable presence in my life.

Toiling with the stick in the laundry ringer, scrubbing and waxing the kitchen floor, dangling a ball over my lazy eye, splashing water in my face after I wet the bed and sprinkling countless heart-shaped *RED HOTS* on my birthday cakes were all beatitudes of kindness not forgotten. While appreciating that my mom gave me the gift of life and enjoying a life I would re-gift, I struggled in finding the perfect gift for her ultimate sentimental journey to Heaven.

Remembering that *the greatest gift you'll ever learn is just to love and be loved in return,* the gift needed to be heartfelt with a note bearing my mother's formal closing of *all my love.* Many years ago she stitched a pair of pillowcases and quilted a blanket to provide comfort to me throughout life. Poignantly, I will return one of these pillowcases for her head to rest upon when she transitions from this life. She and I will share an abiding union that bids sweet dreams and memories for eternity.

As a young child I remember kneeling with my siblings for bedtime prayers. The litany of people to bless always began with *God bless Mommy.* This hopefully places her at the top of St. Peter's list. Little did I realize at that time God had blessed me with a blessed mother who continues to intercede on my behalf and less on my behind. I remain forever grateful to my mother, taking comfort in her resurrection as Mary Anastasia. Happy Birthday, Mom!

All my love.

APPENDIX II

March 24, 2011

MY DEAR DAD

My dad's truth marches on with the precision of a military unit, a well-oiled machine that is designed and drilled to perform at maximum efficiency. Nonetheless, time does cause various parts to break down. Machines utilize the mechanism of synergy, meaning the whole is greater than the sum of its parts. Synergy is synonymous with my dad's career as a mechanic. The sum total of his livelihood has provided countless blessings to me:

> When I was hungry, you gave me "3 squares" to eat.
> When I was thirsty, you gave me "Hi-C" to drink.
> When on a sickbed, you made me walk to school.
> When I was naked, you handed me Ed's clothes
> When I needed direction, you set the example.
> When I was a stranger, you welcomed me home
> saying, "What's up, Doc?"

My inheritance is revealed through the calluses on Dad's hands . . . the ability to diagnose and repair breakdowns while taking pride in his accomplishments. Well-rubbed with Corn Huskers Lotion, his hands opened the wallet virtually tucked in his heart. This lesson of charity was noticeably passed down to me as I open my wallet in support of others. I emulate my dad in being a man of few words. Nevertheless, I needed to find appropriate words to pay tribute to my dad's birth and his life with a gift of thanksgiving.

I treasure the still-life image and memory of Dad's wallet brimming with his children's photos as it rested next to his keychain on the kitchen counter. These keys represented security and transportation provided throughout my childhood. Dad feels rewarded when a paycheck is rendered. Therefore, it seemed appropriate to give my dad a wallet chock-full of money along with a photo of him and me to warm his heart and safeguard his final journey with wishes for many happy returns.

To honor my dad's life includes remembering his service in the armed forces. As a monthly remembrance, I donate to the Wounded Warrior Project that empowers veterans. Future contributions will also be made in gratitude for his unforgotten service in the Korean War and for the salvation of his soul. Warriors aspire to victory. Dad's victory is revealed, revered and remembered by his many loving acts of service and kindness, including the covert routine maintenance performed on my car. Love continues to evolve through transition, but is never forgotten.

My dad's truth marches on as his legs fail to offer him certainty and stability. His inspiring faith contemplates a prime rib banquet in Heaven following an industrious and successful life. Through farming and stewardship, Dad will hopefully reap what he has sown. I envision Dad's celestial kingdom as having bins overflowing with the finest wheat, corn, green beans and tomatoes imaginable. The bread of life and fruit of the vine provided to me in life is certain to sustain my dad in God's favor, blessing him forever. The pride I feel in being Martin's son sustains me with gratitude for all that he has done.

I love you.

APPENDIX III

Will To Die

(Affidavit for Compassionate End-of-Life Care)
Kevin J. Haselhorst, MD

Whereas a terminal condition in its broadest definition leads to death, I underscore and accept that the experience of living will naturally progress to a time to die and my life will end. As defined in the practice of medicine, a terminal condition is an incurable and irreversible illness that leads to death. While treatable medical conditions exist within incurable illness and might be treated for a long period of time in order to prolong life, I would respectfully decline any intervention that might prevent terminal illness from ending my life, particularly while mentally incompetent or unconscious.

Incurable and irreversible illness include: end-stage heart, lung, kidney, and liver disease; diabetes, overwhelming infection, HIV-related illness, most forms of cancer and neurological illness such as stroke, ALS, Alzheimer's and Parkinson's disease. The hallmark of this WILL TO DIE emphasizes my desire to die naturally and gives respect to incurable illness actually assisting in my death. Moreover, I define a terminal condition as being an insufferable and irreversible existence whereby I am unable to live semi-independently following a three-month period of treatment or rehabilitation.

Potentially enduring a terminal condition and incurable illness will justify the personal resolve to have my life end. In lieu of prolonging the time to die, my apparent demise would free me to decline ongoing life-sustaining care in conjunction with the survival rule of threes: 30 minutes of CPR if initiated, three hours on life support if declared brain dead, three days in an intensive care unit, three weeks of hospitalization or three months residing in a long-term care facility. If my recovery lapses while in an unconscious or semiconscious state, I am not to be transferred to a higher level of care.

My living will recognizes that personal dignity and sanctity of life is to be respected, secured with the blessings of free choice, self-determination and the realization that death is an inherent, inevitable and inalienable birthright. As such, I choose to honor the significance and responsibility of being able to decide and declare autonomously whether the quality of my life remains worth living. This WILL TO DIE provides the necessary documentation that advocates my intention to die of natural causes when a terminal condition is present and quality of life becomes mired in total dependency. This WILL TO DIE intends to enshrine my humanity in the midst of a terminal condition.

Any living will is drawn from mindful conviction and heartfelt wishes. My three wishes are *give me liberty or give me death, respect my dignity by allowing me free choice and show me the mercy.* Illness and dying may cause my mind to waver as my body deteriorates. While dying, I may be vulnerable to righteous claims, coercion and tactics that undermine my WILL TO DIE. As a conscientious objector to having life sustained indefinitely, I respectfully wish to silence and absolve those who may feel legally obliged to inform or persuade me with offers of life support. My WILL TO DIE abides in the truth that there is a time to live and a time to die, given by my own terms as outlined.

My end-of-life plan allows me to envision transcending peacefully from this life while lying in the solemn state of levitation. I wish to leave this world unattached to any machines, tubes, lines, infusions or fluids; a simple saline lock will suffice in order to administer sedation. For those who honor my time to die through nurturing and lifting my mind, body and spirit, I commend a similar blessing to their lives and deaths. My WILL TO DIE ultimately provides a prayer for peace and a more universal appeal to encourage others to have their own "wishes to die for" during a time to die.

Kevin J. Haselhorst, MD

APPENDIX IV

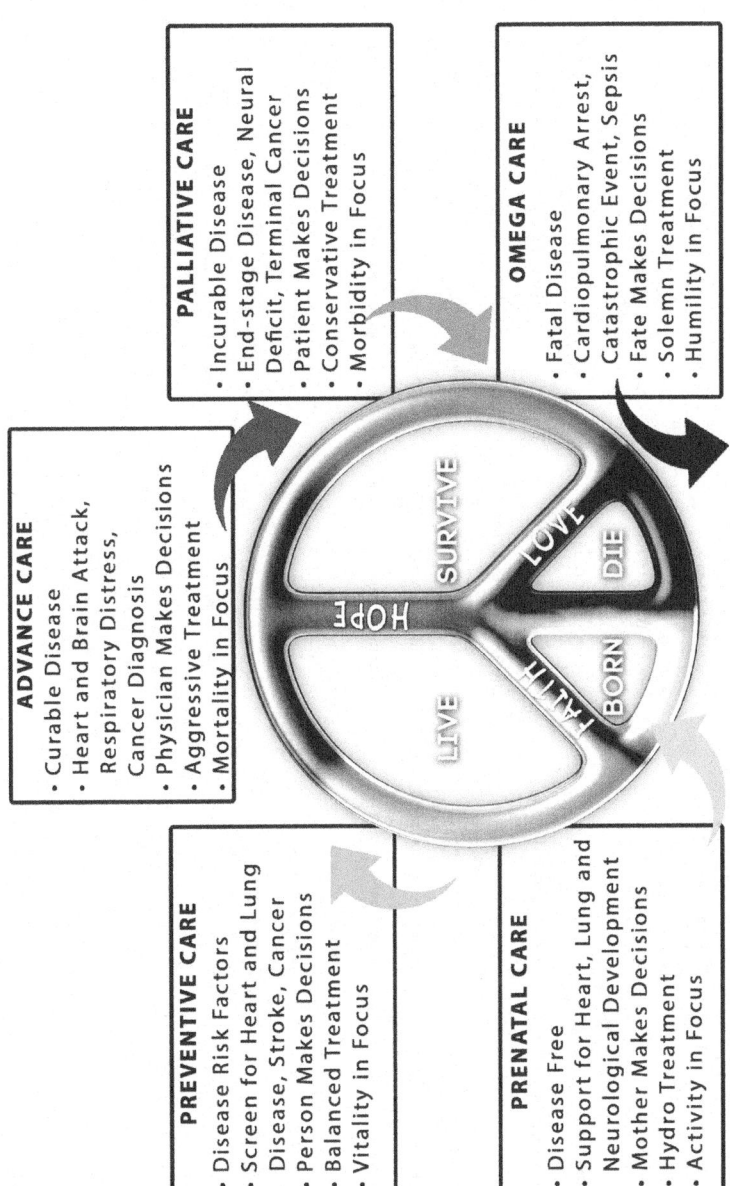

ADVANCE CARE
- Curable Disease
- Heart and Brain Attack, Respiratory Distress, Cancer Diagnosis
- Physician Makes Decisions
- Aggressive Treatment
- Mortality in Focus

PALLIATIVE CARE
- Incurable Disease
- End-stage Disease, Neural Deficit, Terminal Cancer
- Patient Makes Decisions
- Conservative Treatment
- Morbidity in Focus

OMEGA CARE
- Fatal Disease
- Cardiopulmonary Arrest, Catastrophic Event, Sepsis
- Fate Makes Decisions
- Solemn Treatment
- Humility in Focus

PREVENTIVE CARE
- Disease Risk Factors
- Screen for Heart and Lung Disease, Stroke, Cancer
- Person Makes Decisions
- Balanced Treatment
- Vitality in Focus

PRENATAL CARE
- Disease Free
- Support for Heart, Lung and Neurological Development
- Mother Makes Decisions
- Hydro Treatment
- Activity in Focus

SURVIVE

LOVE

DIE

HOPE

FAITH

BORN

LIVE

PRENATAL CARE	PREVENTATIVE CARE	ADVANCE CARE	PALLIATIVE CARE	OMEGA CARE
Disease Free	Disease Risk Factors	Curable Disease	Incurable Disease	Fatalistic Disease
Support for Heart, Lung and Neurological Development	Screen for Heart and Lung Disease, Stroke, Cancer	Heart and Brain Attack, Respiratory Distress, Cancer Diagnosis	End-stage Disease, Neurological Deficit, Terminal Cancer	Cardiopulmonary Arrest, Catastrophic Event, Opportunistic Infection
A Time to be Born	A Time to Live	A Time to Survive	A Time to Let Go	A Time to Die
Anticipation of Life	Engagement in Life	No Retreating from Life	Time to Say Goodbye	Forever Hold Your Peace
Blessed Moment	Life is a Blessing	Life Remains a Blessing	Life is a Mixed Blessing	Death is a Blessing
Conceived Dignity	Explorative Dignity	Assertive Dignity	Nebulous Dignity	Transcendent Dignity
Genetic Engineering	Patient Appointments	Accidental Patient	Perpetual Patient	Patient Unplugged
Sleeping Baby	Person Processes Info	Competent Patient	Semi-Competent Patient	Transitioning Person
Mother Makes Decisions	Person Makes Decisions	Physician Makes Decisions	Patient Makes Decisions	Fate Makes Decisions
Hydro Treatment	Balanced Treatment	Aggressive Treatment	Conservative Treatment	Solemn Treatment
Nurture versus Nature	Nutrition and Exercise	Surgical Candidate	Medical Treatment Only	Comfort Measures only
Womb	Avoid Hospital Admission	ICU Admission	Hospital Admission	Home Environment
Health is a Prayer	Enjoy Health	Reclaim Health	No Claim to Health	Health becomes Non-issue
Activity in Focus	Vitality in Focus	Mortality in Focus	Morbidity in Focus	Humility in Focus
Suffering as Divine Undertaking	Suffering not an Option	Suffering Endured for improvement	Suffering Endured to Live	Cessation of Suffering
Full of Possibility	Full of Potential	Full of Energy	Full of Wonder	Full of Grace
Love Abounds	Faith abounds	Faith Transitions to Hope	Hope Transitions to Love	Love Abounds
Batter-up / Equinox	1st Base / Spring	2nd Base / Summer	3rd Base / Fall	Home Plate / Winter

ABOUT THE AUTHOR

His passion is to transform end-of-life experiences
from catastrophic emergencies to graceful departures.

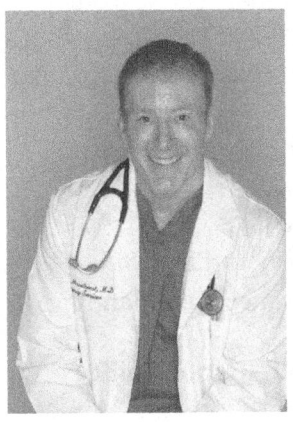

Dr. Kevin Haselhorst grew up in Trenton, Illinois, with dreams of becoming a doctor. Dedication and hard work culminated with a degree in medicine from Southern Illinois University. His residency training at Mercy Hospital in St. Louis opened the doors to the unending excitement of a privileged career in emergency medicine.

Following his tenure in St. Louis, Dr. Haselhorst relocated to Arizona in 1998 and practices at Abrazo Heath hospitals. He is a contributing writer for *The Arizona Republic*'s "Ask the Expert" column, an end-of-life counselor, and a public speaker on Advance Care Directives and the Universal Healthcare Directive.

Dr. Haselhorst blogs on websites for *Wishes To Die For, KevinMD, The Conversation Project* and *Death Café*. He has spoken to caregiver support groups, senior living communities, healthcare provider conferences and church gatherings. He is interviewed regularly on radio and TV.

Follow Dr. Haselhorst . . .
Facebook.com/wishestodiefor
Twitter.com/ wishestodiefor
Linkedin.com/KevinHaselhorst
YouTube.com/KevinHaselhorst

Contact Dr. Haselhorst . . .
DrH@KevinHaselhorst.com
KevinHaselhorst.com

KEYNOTE SPEAKER

A leading voice for compassionate end-of life care, Dr. Haselhorst speaks to individuals, organizations and institutions that are dedicated to personal well-being, lenient healthcare delivery and spiritual awareness during the time to die. End-of-life conversation requires preparation, determination and resolution similar to the principles he brings to his various speaking engagements.

Dr. Haselhorst is a sought-after speaker for:

Caregivers—<u>Insightful</u> Medical Perspective
- Emergency Preparedness: What to Think, Say and Do
- *Wishes To Die For:* Three Milestones to Advance Care Planning

Civic Organizations—<u>Empowering</u> Personal Responsibility
- Healthy, Conscious End-of-life Choice
- ER Doc's Perspective on End-of-Life Blind Spots

Spiritual Communities—<u>Enlighten</u>ed End of Life Pathway
- Amazing Grace: Essential to Dying with Dignity
- Yoga Evokes Stillness at the End of Life

Healthcare Students and Providers—<u>Engaging</u> Patient Spirituality
- One Universal Healthcare Directive
- Medical Breakthroughs of Barriers to Death

"Thank you for having Dr. Haselhorst. He is so knowledgeable and well spoken. He knows the topic well and presents an insight belying his age."
Gateway End-of-Live Conference, St Louis

Have Dr. Haselhorst Speak at Your Event
Visit **KevinHaselhorst.com** or email DrH@KevinHaselhorst.com

THE MISSION

**Life is a journey deserving
of Graceful Departures™**

Kevin Haselhorst, MD

Dr. Kevin Haselhorst is on a quest to change the fear-based perception of dying to this passage becoming an uplifting destination vacation of a lifetime. Graceful Departures™ offers the ways and strategies to approach death and dying with ease and tranquility

Additional insights and resources are available at
Gracefuldepartures.com.

Coordinating a stepwise approach to the end-of-life journey
is necessary for individuals as well as healthcare providers and family
members. An introduction to the thought-process is provided through
Sail the 7 C's of Graceful Departures. This free book is available
at gracefuldepartures.com:

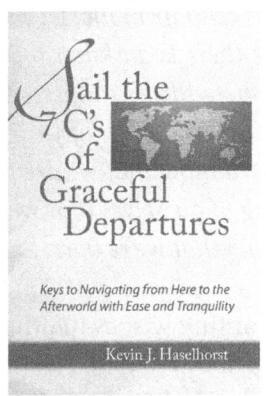

The Share-A-Wish Fund

A gift is a manifestation of the heart
Wishes arise from the depths of the heart

Wishes To Die For

Encourages readers
to have a spiritual
awakening by declaring
and documenting their
heartfelt wishes.

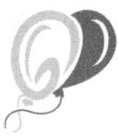

Share-A-Wish Fund

Promotes the universal
power of a wish and
supports children's
charities that make wishes
come true.

Having written *Wishes To Die For* and granting these wishes to others,
I have personified the prayer of St. Francis:

Make me a channel of your peace.
Where there's despair in life, let me bring hope.
Where there is darkness only light,
And where there's sadness ever joy.
Make me a channel of your peace.
It is in pardoning that we are pardoned;
In giving of ourselves that we receive,
And in dying that we're born to eternal life.

In further support of granting wishes to others, a portion of the proceeds from *Wishes To Die For* is gifted to the Share-A-Wish Fund.

More information regarding the Share-A-Wish Fund is available at
wishestodiefor.com

CPSIA information can be obtained
at www.ICGtesting.com
Printed in the USA
FSOW03n0920230316
18168FS